Yourfitnessuccess.com

Functional exercise for seniors

Daily exercise routines for stability, balance, strength & mobility

James Atkinson

Copyright © 2022 yourfitnesssuccess.com

All rights reserved.

CONTENTS

Preface 1
Section 1 3
What is functional exercise? 4
Ageing successfully 8
Basic body mechanics 15
Useful exercise tools 18
Making a functional exercise plan 22
Workouts 28
Range of movement exercise routine 29
Seated exercise routine 33
Single muscle exercise routine 37
Multi muscle exercise routine 41
More daily exercise plans 45
Your exercise routine 51
Section 2 53
Introduction to section 2 54
Range of movement exercises 56
Seated Exercises 74
Single movement exercises 92
Multi movement exercises 118
Thank you! If you found this useful I'd like to help further… 150
Cardio training. 152
Also by James Atkinson 156
Blank workout cards 158

Preface

I want to address the word "senior" as a priority in this book. Technically, if you are over thirty-eight years of age, living in the US and UK, you are on the senior side of the average population. Fitness levels vary immensely from person to person regardless of age. I know twenty-year-olds that would lose fitness related competitions to some sixty, seventy and even eighty-year-olds I also have acquaintances with.

In my experience, age is better represented as a number rather than a condition. It's what we do with our time and how we use our body that makes the difference.

I have also had the privilege of sharing fitness success journeys with people that have been introduced to weight loss and exercise while they were classed as seniors, and, honestly, this has been a highlight of my career as a fitness professional.

As we mature, we find physical exercise more challenging than we would have done in our teens or twenties for several reasons, which will be explained in later chapters, but working on, and maintaining muscle function is something we can all heavily rely on to help us stay flexible, mobile, strong and healthy. Learning to move our bodies in the right way can have an enormously positive impact on our quality of life. This statement is correct for all ages.

My name is James Atkinson (or "Jim" to my readers and friends). I'm a long-term fitness enthusiast of over 25 years with formal, advanced qualifications as a fitness instructor. I have always payed special attention to body mechanics, exercise technique and muscle function to ensure effective, safe exercise sessions, and I firmly believe that any resistance training goal should have roots in the understanding of functional training.

Everyone is different, however, we all have certain weaknesses due to wear and tear, the ageing process in general or previous injury. The exercises in this book are set out as a guide to highlight the movements of the body as they were intended. Some exercise movements may be difficult or may not even be an option, but working with what we have to the best of our ability is all we can do. If you are in doubt or feel that you have a restriction with certain planes of movement that could be improved, a good physiotherapist will be an excellent adviser on a personal level. So if you have pain during any exercise and are unsure why, a session with a physiotherapist could be very valuable.

With all of this said, whatever your age and whatever your fitness level is, there is always a place for functional and mobility training.

Section 1

What is functional exercise?

What is functional exercise? The most basic way to answer this question is with the following statement:

"Functional exercise is moving the body as per its design"

We all know that legs bend at the knees, hips rotate, arms bend at the elbows, etc. But a few examples of less common knowledge are that rounded shoulders are often caused by a weakness in the rear shoulder and upper back muscles and simple activities like sitting down on a chair can strengthen the legs and glute muscles. There are many more examples of everyday activities that we don't think about and take for granted that could be mentioned here, but by the end of this guide, these will become very clear.

With a basic knowledge of body mechanics, we can all drastically change our fitness levels and muscle strength simply by performing everyday activities. Functional fitness is a general term, but I would suggest that it is broken down into a few elements - Range of motion, Balance and muscle strength. Each of these elements can be prioritised, but they all fit together and the benefits of each one overlap.

Range of motion

Range of motion is something that I make a point to highlight in every fitness guide I've written, and part of me wants to apologise to any of you that have read my other books, but the other part of me says it can never be mentioned enough! So sorry (not sorry) here I go again ☺ -

Range of motion, or "ROM" walks hand in hand with flexibility. When we perform any exercise, we should aim to work through our full range of movement. Can you straighten your arms, put your arms out to your sides so they are parallel to the floor, and rotate your palms so they are facing directly upwards?

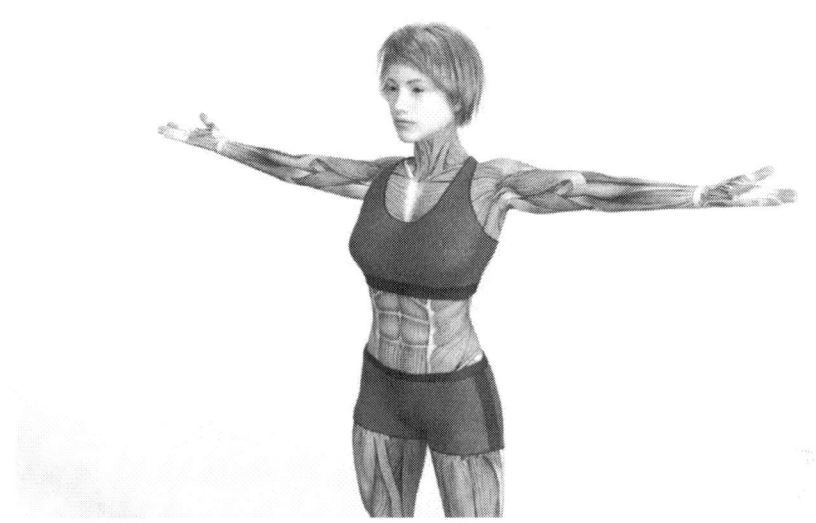

This exercise will test our range of movement in our upper arms, chest, and our shoulder rotation. If this is uncomfortable at all, it may be because these muscle groups are not yet built for a full range of movement. This is very common, so no need to worry. If you struggled with it, we will fix it later in the guide.

Shoulder rotation, arm flexibility and chest opening are just a few examples of upper body range of motion. There is a dedicated set of exercises for range of movement development in section 2 that covers every body part.

Balance

Balance has two meanings with functional fitness; the first is probably the most obvious. Can you stand on one leg with your arms out to your sides without falling over?

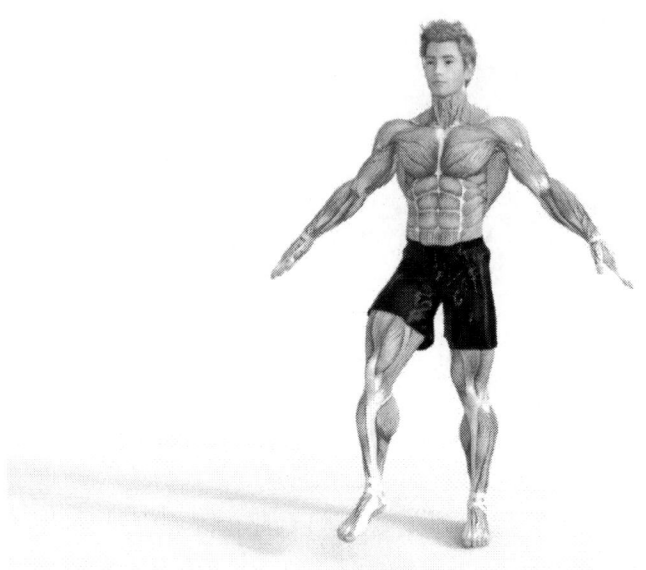

Standing on one leg with your arms out to your sides is a balancing exercise that will engage and challenge a whole range of stabiliser muscles, not just in your legs, but throughout your entire body. The longer you can do this without losing posture or having to put your foot back on the floor, the more these stabiliser muscles will be worked, developing strength and stability.

What's the second meaning of balance then? Can you stand on the other leg with your arms out to your sides for exactly the same time without losing posture or having to put your foot down? There are two sides to the human body and in my experience, we all seem to favour one side over the other. This means that during everyday activities, one side will be used or "developed" and the other, not so much.

Muscle strength

Muscle strength is important, and it's actually one of the main training effects we want to attain by engaging in this type of training in the first place. But if functional fitness is carried out correctly, it will be developed by default.

Any strength exercise that is performed for the first time by a trainer has to be developed. This includes veterans to resistance training. If a trainer has never used barbell squats in their exercise sessions before and they want to start developing leg strength, for example, they would learn the movement with just their bodyweight at first, then gradually add resistance over time, and several training sessions. So the foundation to any muscle strength goal is, in fact, basic muscle function and balance.

Functional fitness training will not give us the type of muscle strength that will help us compete in boulder throwing competitions or ½ tonne deadlifts, but it will give us the muscle strength and function to protect our bones and joints, stay fit, active, flexible and above all longevity all round.

Ageing successfully

As soon as we take our first breath, we are along for the ride. We will all grow and we will all age. There's no getting around it. Studies have been carried out on age and the relation to decline in muscle mass that show we are likely to notice a significant amount of loss in muscle mass at around forty-five years of age. Muscle mass and strength are very important as the more we have, the more protected our bones are. As part of the aging process, our bones also deteriorate and take longer to repair, so having the extra muscle mass will no doubt be extremely beneficial.

During my formal fitness education, my textbooks and mentors told me that after the age of around thirty, we can expect to start losing a small percentage of muscle mass every year. It seems to be common knowledge that as we age, we will deteriorate. And, yes, this is true to some degree, but it is also common knowledge that if we don't challenge our body's functions and muscles, we will also find it increasingly difficult to do so as we age.

"If you don't use it, you'll lose it" is a fantastic phrase that sums up why we should practice functional exercise whatever age we happen to be.

I want to share some real life, personal experience of how this phrase has proven to be correct. I used to train at a gym that had a focus on bodybuilding. This was a warehouse set up on an industrial estate. The gym was basic but well equipped, and most of the members were there to work hard and push themselves. All along the back and sides of the walls, above the huge mirrors, were pictures of members, past and present, that had competed in bodybuilding competitions. These pictures were taken on the day of their shows, so they all looked in fantastic shape!

The age range of the members was fairly wide, but there were plenty of older trainers there, including a guy called Tony. I had seen this guy around the local and in the gym before I actually spoke to him properly, and as soon as I was on general "chit chat" terms, he inspired me pretty much every time we talked. As our acquaintance was workout and gym based, we would talk mostly about training.

Tony was in great shape all the time. He trained with weights most days and was often doing circuit training type workouts or boxing routines on a punch bag. I've always noticed other trainers' exercise form when training in a gym. This is probably because it's something that I take a particular interest in, but Tony had great form and range of movement in everything he did.

During one of our chats, I had asked him how long he had been training for. He said it's something that he always did and always would. It's always tricky asking someone how old they are and I never like to do this but he offered the information without prompt when he told me he was thinking he would like to try another bodybuilding show.

He said something like:

"I'll have to compete in the veteran's category because I'm closer to sixty than I am fifty".

I've always pushed myself when working out and always aimed to be better than I am, so there was no destination. My mentality was that I could always be better. But after Tony had said this, and I had a chance to think about it, I realised that the destination for me was to get well into my senior years and still be in as good a shape as him. This revelation took place about ten years previous to the time of writing, and it becomes more relatable and relevant each year. It's a lesson that I won't forget easily.

I don't plan on doing another bodybuilding competition like Tony, but I do plan on always having a workout routine in place that ensures that I maintain and develop functional fitness as a priority. I want to be like Tony!

Tony wasn't in absolutely perfect health either; he had shoulder injuries, knee pain, and had learned some important lessons about his back during his fitness journey, but he still managed to stay strong all over and in great shape overall.

We all have setbacks from time to time, many of us suffer from ailments of some kind and we are, it seems more prone to these as we get older, but as long as we keep a positive mental attitude and work to stay active around any physical issues the best we can, this can make all the difference.

A close family member of mine was seventy-three years of age when she had a fall fracturing her wrist and pelvis. Fracturing any bone is not a good thing, but a pelvis fracture can be an extremely serious injury, especially for someone of this age.

We were all very concerned as she has always been complemented on "looking good for her age", she is always active and very independent. These injuries, however, meant that she couldn't walk, she couldn't travel up any amount of stairs, she couldn't sleep lying down because of the pain, but the biggest issue to her was that she may never dance again!

To her, losing the ability to carry out everyday activities was something that would not happen. Within days of the injury, she was making efforts to stand up straight and try to hold the position for a few seconds before sitting back in the wheelchair.

During the next few weeks, she would be increasing the amount of times she made the journey from the back door of her house to the front door, using a walking frame whilst shuffling her feet along the floor. Soon, she would be travelling up and down the stairs.

We visited fairly often and heard of these positive and progressive updates daily, but it became apparent to me that although she could now get around, she wasn't using the correct function to do so.

We have a good relationship and I can get away with speaking plainly, so explained that although it was excellent news, there are issues with this.

First, the shuffling along the floor to get around is not walking. The knees don't bend and the hips don't flex as they would when walking, meaning that the legs are not functioning as they should and "if you don't use it, you'll lose it". So the muscles that handle the action of walking were going to atrophy and eventually, shuffling, would be the normal thing to do.

I then learned that to travel up and down the stairs, she was sitting on the stairs and using her upper body and good leg to assist her from step to step. This is not walking up the stairs, this is "sitting up the stairs" and it must have taken a fair amount of upper body strength and effort to do this each time.

After sitting down and explaining the function of the hip and legs, running through the "if you don't use it, you'll lose it" theory and armed with the motivation of being able to dance again soon, we made a video of me stepping onto the first step of a flight of stairs. This was broken down into stages:

Stage 1 – Stand at the bottom of the stairs, ready to climb. Make sure your weight is evenly distributed over both feet.

Stage 2 – shift your weight to your good leg

Stage 3 – Lift your bad leg (the side the pelvis was fractured) to bend it at the knee

Stage 4 – Slowly move this leg forward to place it onto the step

Stage 5 – Transfer your weight from your good leg to the leg on the step

Stage 6 – Push through the foot on the step and straighten your knee

Stage 7 – Bring the other foot up to the step and evenly distribute your body weight again

Stage 8 – Reverse the process

As it was broken down into stages, she could progress through them to the point where it became too tough or exhausting and then try again another day.

By consistently going through this process, several times daily, she was walking up flights of stairs again correctly in less than two weeks. We were all absolutely amazed and pleased by her recovery.

I've always believed that her recovery speed was fuelled by her state of mind; ambition had a huge part in this success story. These days, she does daily dog walks, regular camping trips and, of course, she dances!

If you have had setbacks like this, it's worth seeing a good physiotherapist; they can take you through a similar process to help your recovery. I'm not trained in this field, so when I give advice like this to people, I always have them check it is safe before they go ahead with the plan. More often than not, I find that I'm a bit too cautions with the intensity of the exercises, so recovery should be a lot quicker under a highly trained physiotherapist.

Regular functional exercise and understanding how our muscles and joints are supposed to move goes a long way when it comes to aging successfully. There are, however, other things we should do like eating nutritious food as part of a balanced diet and adding resistance to our workouts.

Resistance training becomes more important as we get older because of the reasons mentioned in the opening of this chapter, and working with resistance is the next progression from range of movement training.

Once we have good range of movement, we can then apply this to resistance training. An example of this is the "shoulder reach" exercise (outlined in this book), when a good range of movement is attained, can be upgraded to "shoulder press". Shoulder press movements can be performed with exercise bands, dumbbells or barbells. Resistance bands, however, are by far the most accessible form of resistance equipment available.

A set of resistance bands is an excellent substitute for barbells and dumbbells for home workouts as they take up hardly any space, are very inexpensive, and if you know how to use them, you have a full gym that will fit into a small bag.

If you are interested in stepping up your training and working on strength and stability, I have created a "follow along" style video course that shows you exactly how to work with resistance bands in your own home to maximum effect. This is a six-week progressive course which includes cardio training as well. There is a big focus on exercise form with each movement we use, so it works in great synergy with this guide.

Follow the link below or type it into your browser if you would like to find out more.

YourFitnessSuccess.com

Home   About   Blog   Podcast   Frequently Asked Questions   Contact   Member Login

Online Home Workout Courses

Fitness results you can count on!

No gimmicks, no fads, just real advice with results in mind.

Let's do this!

START THE COURSE FOR FREE

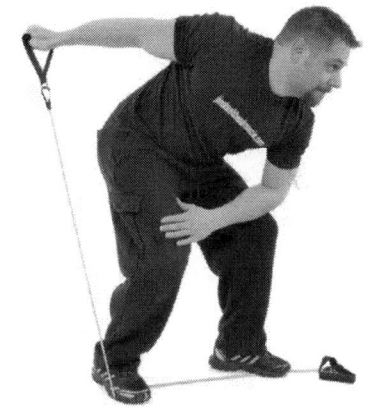

What do others think about this course?

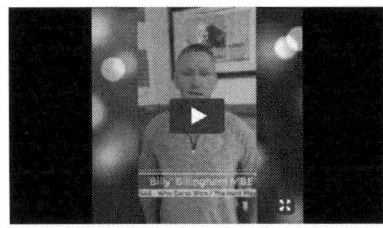
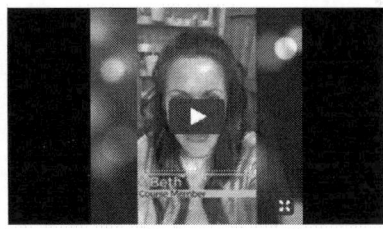

"Far more than your usual fitness video training! This is a serious, progressive exercise course!"

Scan to find out more

As always, I'm happy to answer questions about this and help determine if it is the right move for you. This type of training is not appropriate for everyone, or it might be that range of movement training needs to be practiced for a bit longer before starting something like this. But check it out, we might be training together really soon!

Basic body mechanics

As mentioned earlier, understanding body mechanics is important for functional fitness. By simply moving each body part through its range of motion, we are working on developing function in that area.

Practicing these movements is beneficial to all of us as we will be using our body for what it was designed to do. This is where functional fitness starts.

Each joint in the body is movable to some degree. There are several classifications and sub classifications of joint. This information might be useful as a reference, but knowing all of these terms is not vital for good progression with functional training, and this guide aims to prioritise the most practical and actionable information. Some trainers, however, might find this useful, but to keep it simple, here are the joints and classifications that are most relevant to us, as functional trainers.

Plane joint

Hinge joint

Ball and socket joint

Condyloid

Pivot

Facet

- Ankle – Plane
- Knee – Hinge
- Hip – Ball and socket
- Wrist – Condyloid
- Elbow – hinge
- Shoulder – Ball and socket
- Neck – Pivot
- Spine – Facet

Core function

Core stability and the importance of exercising your core muscles is something that's mentioned by most fitness professionals, and the subject is often seemingly an afterthought when exercise movements are described or demonstrated.

Before performing any exercise, be it a barbell squat or a seated leg lift, there should always be a "setup" with body position and an understanding about what the exercise is designed to achieve.

I have always believed that the setup before an exercise is as important as the exercise itself. If we take the time to set ourselves up for every movement sufficiently enough, the exercise will not only be more productive and efficient, but it will help to guard against injury whilst also strengthening our overall posture.

Pretty much every exercise that we perform has an engagement of our core muscles. Lower back and abdominals are the basic terms for our core. As part of the setup for any exercise described in this guide, we should always engage our abdominals and glutes to some degree.

Abdominals

To engage the abdominals, we don't have to go into a full crunch, as this would be counterproductive. The easiest way to get this engagement is to take a deep breath, slowly exhale and at the point that your lungs are nearly empty, you will feel your abdominals tighten slightly. Hold this abdominal position and continue breathing normally. It may take a bit of practice, but this is something that can be tested whilst sitting in a chair.

Once you have this abdominal engagement perfected, maintain it throughout your sets and reps of your exercises.

Lower back

The breathing technique to engage the abdominals will also engage the lower back slightly, but this is normally not enough. Because the lower back muscles are not as easy to engage as other muscles, we can use the glutes to help this. The glute muscles are part of what is known as "the posterior chain". The posterior chain is basically all the muscles that run up the back of the body, but we are interested in engaging our lower back.

If we tense our glutes, this activates the lower back muscles called the "erector spinae". Learning how to engage our glutes from my experience is best to practice from a standing position. Stand with your feet about shoulder width apart, make sure your back is straight and simply push your hips forward without moving your upper body, this should fire your glutes up, hold the tension for a few seconds before returning to the start position and repeat. Once you can do this comfortably and have a good mind muscle connection, you can try it from a seated position.

To learn to engage our glutes from a seated position is a bit more difficult and I would suggest if you can, learn to do it from the standing position mentioned above. This way, you will know what it feels like and simply be able to "clench your glutes. If standing is not an option for you, try this: Sit on a seat with your back supported, place both feet on the floor close to the legs of the chair. Keep your back flat and engage your abdominals.

From this position, push through your heels as if you were trying to lift your whole body off the chair. If your setup position is good, you will not actually move from the chair, but your hamstrings will fire first, then your glutes should engage.

If you follow these abdominal and glute engagement steps as part of your setup prior to every exercise movement, it will soon become second nature and you will be working on core stability and strength by default during everything you do.

Useful exercise tools

Working against gravity and moving our body through its range of motion are the most accessible forms of exercise, but as we all know, there are plenty of ways to increase the challenge by adding resistance to our exercise movements and there are also ways to aid us with progression with fuller range of motion.

Most of the exercises in this book are illustrated as bodyweight movements

Support

The "one leg balance" is a good example of an exercise that may require a support. Not everyone will be able to go right into this movement without some conditioning, so using a support for the development of this exercise is a great way to start. In this case, a support could be any stable object, such as a wall or chair. The idea of using a support is not to rely on it for the movement, it is there to aid us with our balance so we can hold the position for longer, and therefore develop our muscle strength in order to progress away from needing the support at all.

When using a support for any exercise, we should never use it as a crutch and rest our weight on it or use it for momentum to complete the movement. I find the best way to work with a support is to use only my fingertips to connect myself to the support.

Sticking with the example of the "one leg balance", this is how I would advise using a support:

- Stand with a wall directly to your left.
- Raise your left arm so it is in line with your mid torso and out to your side.
- Side step towards the wall until your fingertips touch it. This now becomes your support position.
- The leg farthest from the wall will be your working leg, so raise your left foot off the floor.

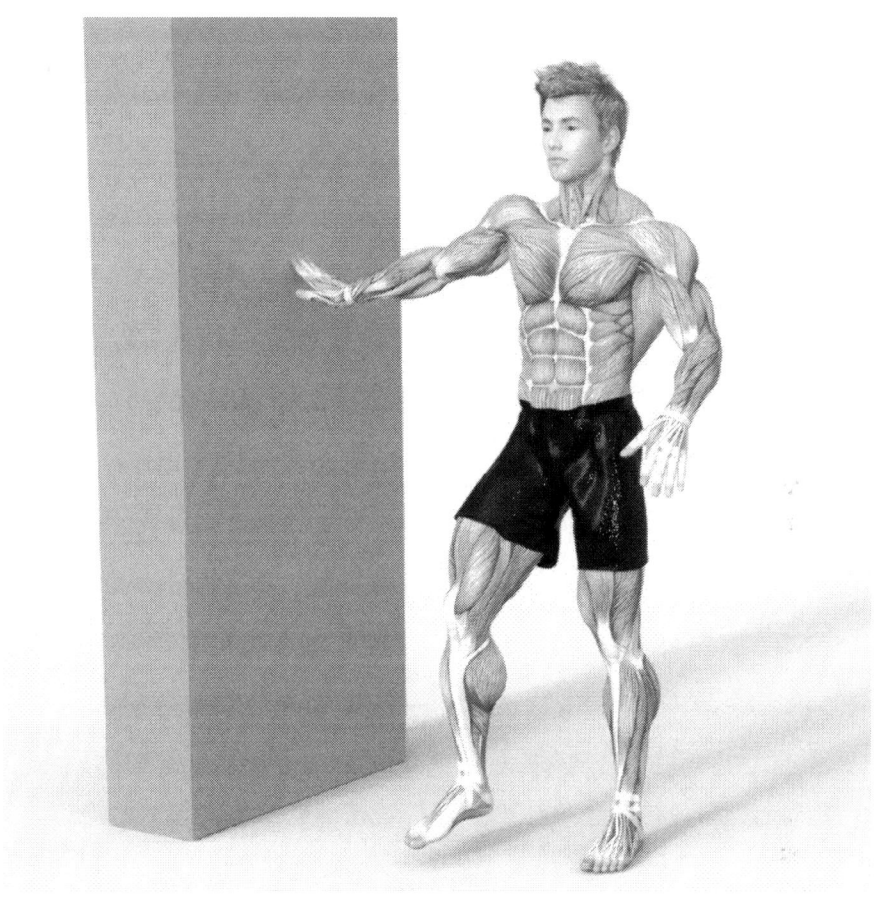

You can choose to use either leg as your working leg, but the reason I suggest using the leg farthest from the support is that the support technically becomes the substitute for the raised leg. Again, this is down to personal preference, so try both and see which is best for you.

You can do this by facing the wall and having your arms out in front of you too, but the fingertip contact should be maintained if you can.

If you practise this consistently, it will not be long before you can lower your hands and keep them by your sides whilst performing this exercise.

To progress from a supported exercise, we should regularly try to move our contact away from the support during our session; this can be for a second or two at a time until we can do our planned exercise fully without its use.

Resistance bands

Resistance bands can be used for rehabilitation, strength building and flexibility. They are available in many variations, and these bits of exercise equipment are useful for everyone. There are plenty of benefits for using resistance bands in our training when it comes to conditioning and muscle development, but as they are relatively inexpensive and compact, this makes them that bit more accessible for most.

Many of the exercises in this book can be adapted to use resistance bands, and I would argue that workouts with resistance bands are the next progression to resistance training from basic bodyweight and mobility. There is a fair bit to be said about training with resistance bands and there are multiple uses and I don't want to drift too far off topic in this book. If you are interested in getting into this type of training, I've written a short beginner's guide as part of this series. You can check out the "Resistance band training" book for a heads up and a few exercises to try.

Weights

Dumbbells, barbells, EZ bars, sandbags, kettlebells, and the list goes on. There are many types of weights out there to train with if you want a specific training effect. As mentioned, adding extra resistance to your exercises sessions is the next progression from bodyweight and mobility exercise. Resistance bands are a good start and often all a trainer will need, as there is plenty of scope for increased exercise intensity and the creation of increasingly challenging workouts with a basic set of bands. But due to the nature of resistance bands, there is a variable resistance increase of resistance through any movement.

As the band stretches, the resistance increases, so the start of the movement will not be as hard as the top of the movement. This is where weights are different.

Performing a bicep curl with a resistance band will see the bicep being stressed the most at its maximum contraction as the resistance band is stretched most at this point, so the exercise will be easier at the start of the movement.

Performing the same bicep curl with a weight such as a dumbbell or barbell (assuming we are using the correct exercise form) will ensure that the resistance level is consistent from the start of the movement right through to the top of the movement.

Barbells and dumbbells come in all sorts of shapes and sizes, but they are worth exploring if you are looking to take resistance training to the next level. As it is with resistance bands, barbell and dumbbell training is a big subject and for beginners with this type of training, there is a lot to understand and practice before effective training sessions can be achieved. But training with these types of weights is absolutely worth investigating.

I have also written a good beginner's guide for barbells and dumbbells if this is something that you might be interested in. You can check out "Barbell & Dumbbell Training" if you want to try this out.

Weights, however, don't have to be heavy discs or iron bars, though. A weight used for resistance training could be anything from bottles of water, tins of beans or you can even invest in small dumbbells weighing fractions of a kilogram or wrist and ankle weighted straps.

I would advise that if you are using household objects that you choose things that have an even weight distribution and are easy to grip. Food tins and some water bottles are good examples.

Making a functional exercise plan

Having the knowledge of how to optimise your body's movement to engage your muscles correctly during everyday activities is a solid start. By simply being aware and attempting to work your muscles in everyday actions, such as sitting on a chair or picking something up from the floor, can have a big impact on functional fitness development, and this may be enough for some people.

However, I'm a big advocate of following a training plan for any type of fitness development. From flexibility to bodybuilding, from long distance running to rehabilitating a single muscle group after an injury, having a plan in place and following it regularly will not only ensure fitness development, but it will help the trainer assess progress.

Functional fitness training does not differ from any other type of training with planning. In this section, we will look at a few different training plan examples you can follow directly or switch up a bit to better fit your goals. At the back of the book, there are some blank training cards so you can have a go at creating your very own plans to follow. This is a resource that I always add into my training books as it's a great opportunity to create a full, bespoke plan that fits directly with your goals, and it's easy to make copies for future upgrades as you progress. Creating and keeping these cards will also give you a record of your progress.

There are countless ways to plan your functional training sessions. The following program card set up is my design. This is by no means the only way to plan your own exercise sessions, but it should give you an idea of some elements of a training that you can consider and track.

Here's an explanation for clarity:

FUNCTIONAL TRAINING

ROUTINE				
EXERCISE		SETS	REPS	TIME

- Your exercise choices here
- Number of sets here
- Name your routine
- Number of repetitions here
- Days of exercise sessions
- Time of exercise here

WEEKS	MON	TUE	WED	THURS	FRI	SAT	SUN
1							
2							
3							
4							
5							

Name your routine

The name of your routine could be anything, as long as you know what it means. In the examples, I've named the routines so that they fit with a goal or fit to a specific type of exercise method. It is possible to create several routines for different body parts or functions and use them on different days. For example, you could create a "dynamic exercise session" and have this for Monday sessions, a "full body compound exercise session" for Wednesday sessions and call them "dynamic Monday" and "compound Wednesday" etc.

If you are starting out, however, I suggest that you follow a single exercise plan from the examples or create your own plan that you simply repeat. This way, it's less overwhelming and you can become proficient at a handful of exercises before moving on.

Your exercise choices here

Your exercise choices are listed in this column. You can choose exercises that target the whole body, a certain muscle group, several muscle groups, and you can even have whole exercise sessions that use multiple exercises for the same muscle group.

Your exercise choices should reflect your current ability and align with your functional training goals. If you struggle to perform certain exercise from a standing position, for example, you should not focus on standing movements, choose seated exercises for your main workload and maybe add some standing movements at the end to challenge yourself for future progression. This way, the bulk of your session is more likely to be of higher quality to the target area or muscle group and any exercises that you might struggle with are seen as a "work in progress".

The number of exercises you choose to add is up to you. But I would suggest choosing a minimum of five and a maximum of ten. A thirty to forty-five minutes of exercise is a good goal, timewise, so it's important to ensure you can fit all you have planned into this timescale. Remember that concentration on the exercises, especially movements that are not familiar, can add to fatigue. I would advise to start off with a conservative number of exercises. If you find you get through these with no time or fatigue issues, simply add another exercise choice to your next session.

Number of sets here

The sets are the amount of times you intend to perform a set number of repetitions of an exercise before having a short rest. With the subject of this guide in mind, I would suggest using between one and three sets of an exercise. Of course, you can choose to increase this number of sets on exercise movements that you feel need more attention.

Number of repetitions here

The number of repetitions (reps) that you plan to perform inside of each set is marked in this column. For this guide, I would suggest performing between eight and fifteen reps per set. You may find some exercise choices more challenging than others, causing you to become fatigued and lose good exercise form. As we already know, exercise form is very important, so if, for example, you planned to perform ten reps of an exercise but can only manage five before losing form, just make a note of how many reps you actually managed to complete in the box and aim to beat it next time. This is another benefit of having a working program card.

Time of exercise here

If you plan on working with sets and reps exclusively, this column can be ignored, but there are some exercise choices that work better with "time performed" rather than how many times you perform it. Examples of these exercises are static movements, such as the single leg balance and range of movement exercises. With "timed exercises," it may be that the time performing an exercise is dictated by your strength or ability to perform the exercise. The one leg balance, for example, might be very challenging for some trainers, causing fatigue after a second or two. If this is the case for you, simply perform the exercise for as long as you can and make a note in the "time" column next to this particular exercise. You can aim to beat it next time.

Timed training can be used for every exercise. As long as the exercise form is on point and it is performed with control, you can choose to run all of your chosen exercises within a time frame rather than counting the reps. I would suggest that this is a progression from the "sets and reps" training method, however as in my experience, it can dilute the concentration causing exercise technique to suffer.

Days of exercise sessions

Choosing which days to do your exercise session on is important. If you do not have this planned out, and an "exercise slot" allocated to your day from week to week, it's very easy to miss out. Exercise progression comes from regular, consistent exercise, whatever your training goal is. This is why I've included this section on the program card.

Once you have your routine planned out, consider your lifestyle and try to work your exercise sessions around it. If you are new to exercise, training three times per week is a good start. Pick three none consecutive days to train on and stick to this for a few weeks to test the water. The reason for none consecutive training days is to give your body chance to recover. It may be that you are able to move up to more regular training sessions quickly. Depending on your exercise choices, exercise intensity, and how quickly you recover, you may soon find that your exercise sessions become part of your daily routine.

As functional training methods are designed to focus on joint and muscle function, flexibility and range of motion, this type of training lends itself well to daily training routines, and this should be your goal, but everyone has a different set of circumstances and are at different levels of fitness. Listen to your body. If you need a rest day, take one.

The blank program cards

I always encourage readers of my fitness guides to work on creating their own exercise programs as this helps to make training sessions more specific and therefore more valuable to readers than using one of the example routines in the book. Photocopying a blank card from the paperback version or even writing directly into the book is far better than having a digital version, in my opinion. This is because you can write notes onto the card, strike-through and update without having it stored out of sight on a digital device. Call me old-fashioned, but in my experience, this works.

Your exercise card doesn't have to be clean. As long as you know what it means and you can see your progress, it's good enough.

I enjoy hearing from people who have read my guides and are more than happy to help where I can, so if you have any questions about setting up your routine, drop me an email, I'll do my best to help you get on track where I can. Also, if you need a PDF copy of the blank program card, I'll happily send you one over.

Workouts

In the next part of this guide, we'll look at a few examples of exercise routines that can be performed and several different methods of how to train or utilise the exercises.

All the following routines can be tweaked to fit with your personal set of circumstances, so if you would like to follow one of these routines, but find one or more of the exercises within the routine to difficult, you can simple miss it out or switch it for another exercise of your choice. However, keep in mind that your exercises choices and methods should align with your training goals. For example, if your training goal is to increase range of movement, it's a good idea to stick to exercises that challenge this area, rather than choosing exercises that are more strength focused.

With that said, any exercise choice that is performed with good form and challenges you physically is beneficial, but if you can identify your weaknesses and work on making them your strengths, the benefits will be even more powerful.

The following exercise routines can be copied and printed out, so if you want to follow one of these routines directly, you actually have a hard copy to make notes on or adjust as you train. In my experience, exercise cards like these are not meant to be pretty; they are always a work in progress and a record of our progression through our exercise journey. So make notes, strike through and highlight things where you need to and when it's time for a new one, keep your old cards to look back on. I've always found this very interesting and sometimes inspirational.

Range of movement exercise routine

The first exercise routine I want to cover has a focus on full body range of movement. In my opinion, range of movement is the most important aspect of fitness that you can work on as it helps with alignment, mobility, posture and with a body that has all over, good range of movement, functional exercises for strength training, balance and even progressions into resistance training will be more easily performed and more effective.

FUNCTIONAL TRAINING

ROUTINE: Range of movement

EXERCISE	SETS	REPS	TIME
Chest opening	3	8	-
Head and neck mobility	3	8	-
Hip rotation	3	8	-
Spinal roll down	3	8	-
Ankle roll	3	8	-
Cat cow	3	8	-
Waist twist	3	8	-

WEEKS	MON	TUE	WED	THURS	FRI	SAT	SUN
1	★		★		★		
2	★		★		★		
3	★		★		★	★	
4	★		★		★	★	
5							

Exercises

As advertised, the exercises in this routine are focused on the development of range of movement. Like all exercises, these are performed with slow control. When performing exercises such as "chest opening", "spinal roll down", "waist twists" and "cat cow", concentrate on a slow smooth movement to the point of your current range. Once you reach the top of movement on these exercises, hold for a few seconds before slowly returning to the start position.

When performing the other exercises: "head and neck mobility", "hip rotation" and "ankle roll", these should also be performed in a slow and controlled manner. Note that "hip rotation" and "ankle roll" are continuous movements, but the "head and neck mobility" exercise has a pause at each position

Sets

I've chosen 3 sets of each exercise, as this is a good starting point for most. However, if you feel that this is too much for you at the moment, there is no issue in dropping the sets to 2 or even 1 on exercises that you struggle with. Note that some exercises require multiple movements and some are performed on each limb. Exercises such as "ankle roll" should have a set dedicated to each ankle, so even though it states "3 sets of ankle roll", you would perform 3 sets on each ankle.

Reps

The rep range on this routine is set at 8 reps per exercise. For this range of movement exercise routine, I have chosen 8 reps per exercise as this rep range will challenge most of us suitably. If the 8 rep range is too challenging on any given exercise, this can be reduced. I would suggest drop to 5 or even 3 reps. The quality of the exercise movement is always more important that the amount of times it is performed.

Note that exercises such as "head and neck mobility" have multiple movements and stages, so a single rep is a full rotation. This is explained with more clarity in the exercise description in section 2.

Time

As we are working with sets and reps, we are not using a timed workout, so this column is not applicable in this particular exercise routine.

Training days

When starting a new exercise routine, it is sensible to let our body recover before it is challenged again. I've chosen a three day per week training pattern for the first two weeks and then added an extra training day for the third and fourth week. You will notice that each training day in the first two week pattern is also placed on non-consecutive days, so there is a rest day between workouts. Although functional training like this can be performed daily, if our bodies are not used to it, they can become fatigued, so a gentle increase like this is always advised for beginners.

Again, this is a work in progress and if you feel after the first week that you can do more, plan to exercise on more days by marking your program card.

Seated exercise routine

This seated exercise routine is designed to work through the major muscle groups to promote function with mobility, range of movement and a degree of muscle strengthening.

FUNCTIONAL TRAINING

ROUTINE	**Seated exercise**

EXERCISE	SETS	REPS	TIME
Chest opening	3	10	-
Seated low row	3	10	-
Knee bend	3	10	-
Leg lift – Knee bent	3	10	-
Shoulder reach	3	10	-
Calf raise seated	3	10	-
Seated hip hinge	3	10	-

WEEKS	MON	TUE	WED	THURS	FRI	SAT	SUN
1	*		*		*		
2	*		*		*		
3	*		*		*	*	
4	*		*		*	*	
5							

Exercises

All the exercise descriptions in this routine are available in the "seated exercises" part of section 2 apart from "chest opening". This is listed with the "range of movement" exercises.

The rest of the exercise choices in this routine engage a specific set of muscles, "shoulder reach" targets the shoulder muscles, "seated low row" targets the back muscles etc. an important part of any exercise is the setup and posture held throughout the movement, and seated exercises are no different. When performing seated exercises, you should always ensure that you have a flat back and your core is engaged.

Sets

I've chosen 3 sets of each exercise again. And as before, there's no issue in dropping the sets to 2 on exercises that you struggle with. There's also an option to increase the amount of sets you do for each exercise, but I would suggest not increasing past 4 sets. There are also exercises that are single limb movements. Remember that you will be performing a set on each limb, so these exercises will take double the time.

Reps

The rep range on this routine is set at 10 reps per exercise, but if this is too challenging, again, you can drop the range. With exercises like these, if you need to drop the reps, do so by increments of 2. Increasing the reps is possible in the same way, but I would suggest that 15 is the maximum you climb to. If you feel that you need more from your exercise routine, you can always add exercise choices.

Time

As we are working with sets and reps, we are not using a timed workout, so this column is not applicable in this particular exercise routine.

Training days

This is the same training pattern as the previous routine for the same reasons. Although this is technically a different style of training, the same rules apply when it comes to rest, recovery and, indeed, a steady transition into a training routine.

Single muscle exercise routine

This is an example of a single muscle, timed workout that involves exercises for a range of muscle groups. There is, however, a bigger focus on the upper body. I would class this routine as intermediate level, as the exercises involved may require some prior conditioning before they can be performed effectively.

FUNCTIONAL TRAINING

ROUTINE	**Single muscle**		
EXERCISE	**SETS**	**REPS**	**TIME**
Bicep curls	3	-	20 secs
Tricep extension	3	-	20 secs
Hover sit	3	-	20 secs
Lateral raises	3	-	20 secs
Front raises	3	-	20 secs
Seated crunch	3	-	20 secs
Hip extension	3	-	20 secs

WEEKS	MON	TUE	WED	THURS	FRI	SAT	SUN
1	*		*		*		
2	*		*		*		
3	*		*		*	*	
4	*		*		*	*	
5	*		*	*	*		

Exercises

Most exercises in this routine are based around movements that can be easily upgraded to add resistance, such as small dumbbells, resistance bands and, in some cases a barbell. "Bicep curl", "tricep extension", "lateral raises" and "front raises" all target a single muscle group and they can also be performed from a seated position, but standing with good posture while exercising will add extra value to your workouts.

Sets

3 sets for each exercise again, but as we are working with time on this routine, the sets are a variable that breaks up each exercise only. 3 sets of 20 seconds means we will have a full minute per exercise with 3 short breaks. As you get stronger and more competent at performing exercises like this, you may want to increase the time and drop the sets, or increase both! There is a lot of scope for progression.

Reps

As we are working with time per exercise here, we can ignore the reps column.

Time

I've chosen to start with 20 seconds per set of each exercise. In my experience, this is a good number to open on, as we can easily break this down into 3 sets to give us a full minute on each movement. When working with time slots, it's really important to ensure we maintain a constant and controlled cadence with the exercise movements. For example, when I am training a client, I will count 2 - 3 seconds from the start of the movement to the top of movement and the same on the return, depending on the client's fitness level. This rhythm should be continuous throughout the allotted training time.

As an aside, the exercises in this functional training routine can also be trained with the sets and reps method as per the previous program card (3 sets of 10 reps per exercise). This gives you the option to decide on the day of your workout whether you would like to train with the timed method or in the sets and reps style.

Training days

The training days are the same as the previous routines, but I've shown a progression on week 5 by adding an extra training day. This makes it a 5 day training week. If you decide to change up your routines by making the workouts more intense, however, it may be a bit much to add extra training days, so this is something to be aware of.

Multi muscle exercise routine

This multi muscle, functional exercise routine example challenges the whole body with compound movements and balance and it makes use of timed exercises along with the "sets and reps" training method. There is a lot going on, and I would suggest that this type of exercise routine is for trainers that have developed a good range of movement and a strong foundation of muscle strength.

If you like the look of the following routine, but feel some of the exercises might be out of your reach, you can always allocate some time at the end of your routine to practice the exercise. This is exactly what I have done in my own training with exercises that I've wanted to start incorporating into my workouts, a great way to learn and to progress!

If you are working on range of movement exercises, for example, but would like to learn a "cross leg sit", you can add the exercise to the end of your workout. "The cross leg sit" is set out in stages in the exercise description, like many others, so you can practise one stage at a time.

FUNCTIONAL TRAINING

ROUTINE: **Multi muscle**

EXERCISE	SETS	REPS	TIME
Wall push ups	4	12	-
Pick & lift	3	10	-
Step ups	3	-	30 secs
Over head push	4	12	-
Balance & hip extension	3	-	20 secs
Twist & reach	3	12	-
Cross leg sit	3	-	30 secs

WEEKS	MON	TUE	WED	THURS	FRI	SAT	SUN
1	★		★		★		
2	★		★		★		
3	★		★		★	★	
4	★		★		★	★	
5	★		★	★	★	★	

Exercises

The exercises chosen for this workout routine are all compound movements, meaning they target multiple muscle groups with every rep. This means that each rep requires more effort to perform; furthermore, it means that we also have to concentrate more on body positioning, posture and exercise form.

Sets

The exercises in this routine have either 4 or 5 sets. You can switch up the amount of sets per exercise within a routine. Adding sets to an exercise is done to add a bigger workload to an exercise. This can be done to an exercise that you feel you need more development on or it can be to add intensity to exercises that you are progressing with quicker than others.

Reps

The exercise choices that are marked with reps are performed with 10 or 12 reps. I've chosen to add a different number to some exercises to highlight what's possible when creating your own routine. Some exercises will be a lot tougher than others. This could be down to the nature of the exercise or it could mean that there is a weaker muscle group that the exercise is designed to target. Either way, we should always prioritise exercise technique over workload, so if our form starts to suffer because of fatigue, this is our maximum effort. If this means it's only 3 reps, that's fine, we can try for 4 next time.

Time

This is an exercise program that makes use of time and reps. The exercises that use time in this example are movements that lend themselves to this training method better than they do with the reps method.

"Step ups" simulate the function that our body would use when we step onto an elevated surface, so muscles and joints are put to use for an everyday activity here, but as this is a big movement (depending on the height of the step), we can benefit from a cardio aspect of fitness here too. A continuous compound movement like this can add a dynamic feel to your workouts.

The "cross leg sit" is an exercise that requires a lot of practice for most people, and those who can perform it will benefit from holding good posture in the final seated position. The clock starts when we have completed the transition from standing to seated.

Training days

The training days for this example are the same as the previous routine. Training days can be changed from week to week, but I would suggest that training at least three times per week should be the benchmark.

More daily exercise plans

In this section, you will find several more examples of daily exercise routines to follow directly, or take inspiration from when creating your own. It is possible to use a variety of routines throughout any given week. You could even use a different routine every day, or allocate a certain type of exercise to certain days of the week.

The following plans serve as templates for you to work with. For this reason, the "sets", "reps" and "time" columns will be left blank, along with the "Week" section at the bottom of the card. This is yours to decide how you would like to use it.

On each routine card, there will be an indication of what the workout aims to address. Look out for this in the "Routine" field at the top. Each workout will have a goal.

For some guidance and a general rule to follow on workload: a strong starting point with the sets and reps range on most exercises would be 3 sets of 10 – 15 reps and when using timed exercises, 20 seconds to one minute is usually a good range for most trainers.

FUNCTIONAL TRAINING

ROUTINE	**Balance & upper body ROM**		
EXERCISE	**SETS**	**REPS**	**TIME**
Chest opening			
Head and neck mobility			
Shoulder rotation			
Shoulder reach			
Ankle roll			
Single leg balance			
Leg lift & widening			

WEEKS	MON	TUE	WED	THURS	FRI	SAT	SUN
1							
2							
3							
4							
5							

FUNCTIONAL TRAINING

ROUTINE	Legs and core strength

EXERCISE	SETS	REPS	TIME
Balance & hip extension			
Squats or hover sit			
Good mornings			
Step & reach			
Twist & reach			
Seated crunch			
Dorsal raise			

WEEKS	MON	TUE	WED	THURS	FRI	SAT	SUN
1							
2							
3							
4							
5							

FUNCTIONAL TRAINING

ROUTINE	Arms, shoulders & back			
EXERCISE		SETS	REPS	TIME
Bicep curls				
Tricep extension				
Lateral raises				
Front raises				
Overhead push				
Bent over row				
Pick & lift				
Dorsal raise				

WEEKS	MON	TUE	WED	THURS	FRI	SAT	SUN
1							
2							
3							
4							
5							

FUNCTIONAL TRAINING				
ROUTINE	**Full body, big movements**			
EXERCISE		SETS	REPS	TIME
Wall push or full push ups				
Bent over rows				
Pick and lift				
Shoulder reach				
Bicep curl				
Tricep extension				
Dorsal raise				
Seated crunch				

WEEKS	MON	TUE	WED	THURS	FRI	SAT	SUN
1							
2							
3							
4							
5							

FUNCTIONAL TRAINING

ROUTINE	ROM & Balance		

EXERCISE	SETS	REPS	TIME
Head & neck mobility			
Leg lift & widening			
Shoulder rotation			
Balance & hip extension			
Spinal roll down			
Chest opening			
Cat cow			
Single leg balance			

WEEKS	MON	TUE	WED	THURS	FRI	SAT	SUN
1							
2							
3							
4							
5							

Your exercise routine

Exercise routines are very subjective. Everybody is different. We all have our strengths and weaknesses and differing physical abilities, but if we can identify our problem areas, we can work on progressive, positive development.

If you connected with any of the exercise routine examples and would like to try them as they are, go for it! If you are new to this type of planning or layout, it will more than likely help you get into the groove of a training pattern and give you the starting blocks for your own personalised routine that aligns with your fitness goals.

If you've already skipped to section 2 and seen exercises you would like to work with, that have not been mentioned in the example routines, or you want to design your own program right now, here is a blank card for you to do just that with:

FUNCTIONAL TRAINING

ROUTINE

EXERCISE	SETS	REPS	TIME

WEEKS	MON	TUE	WED	THURS	FRI	SAT	SUN
1							
2							
3							
4							
5							

Section 2

Introduction to section 2

Section 2 is all about the exercises choices. Every exercise has at least two illustrations, along with a written description on how to perform it correctly. Please take the time to read these descriptions, as there are useful tips that simply can't be shown in an image.

It's important to be fully familiar with what an exercise does, so you can get the most value in your training sessions and avoid unnecessary injury.

The exercises choices have been broken down into four categories for ease of selection when it comes to the design of your workout routine.

Range of movement exercises

Range of movement exercises are listed first, as I believe this aspect of fitness should be the foundation of any resistance based, functional training and mobility goal. Although most of these exercises are illustrated showing a standing position, they can be performed from a seated position too.

These exercises can be viewed as "tests" so if you find that you have a limited range of movement in certain areas, you can still move on to some of the other workouts, but I would advise that you add the range of movement test that you struggle with to your regular workouts. These exercises will always be valuable and even if you are confident that you have a perfect range of movement, they are always worth revisiting from time to time.

Seated exercises

Seated exercises are listed next. Standing for prolonged periods can be exhausting, and holding a good posture whilst doing this can be a complete workout in itself for some people. Seated exercise can be a great option for trainers that would like to target muscle groups from a seated position allowing them to focus more on the exercises, rather than running the risk of diluting the movement while concentration is split between standing and actually performing the exercise.

Single muscle exercises

Listed next are the single muscle exercises. As the title suggests, these movements are designed to target single muscle groups, so they have a fairly specific goal. Working single muscle groups will work towards strengthening them individually, so they will perform better with multi muscle movements. For example, working the shoulders with a reach movement, the quads with an extension, the glutes with hip extension, and the lower back with a dorsal raise will work most muscle groups that are required to perform a lift & reach which is a multi-muscle exercise.

Multi-muscle exercises

Last but not least are multi-muscle exercises. These movements are big ones that call upon several muscle groups to complete and can take a lot of concentration to perform correctly. I would class these as more advanced movements. If you are new to exercises, this is something to work up to by becoming comfortable with the range of movement and single muscle exercises first. With that said, if you are a beginner and would still like to try these out anyway, study the exercise, and break it down into sections if you need to before jumping in. Remember that these exercises often require full focus, so concentrate throughout the whole movement.

If you are confident in performing these exercises, you can have a workout plan that uses multi-muscle movements exclusively. But even adding a few of these movements into your workout plan can be a massive upgrade.

Range of movement exercises

Ankle roll

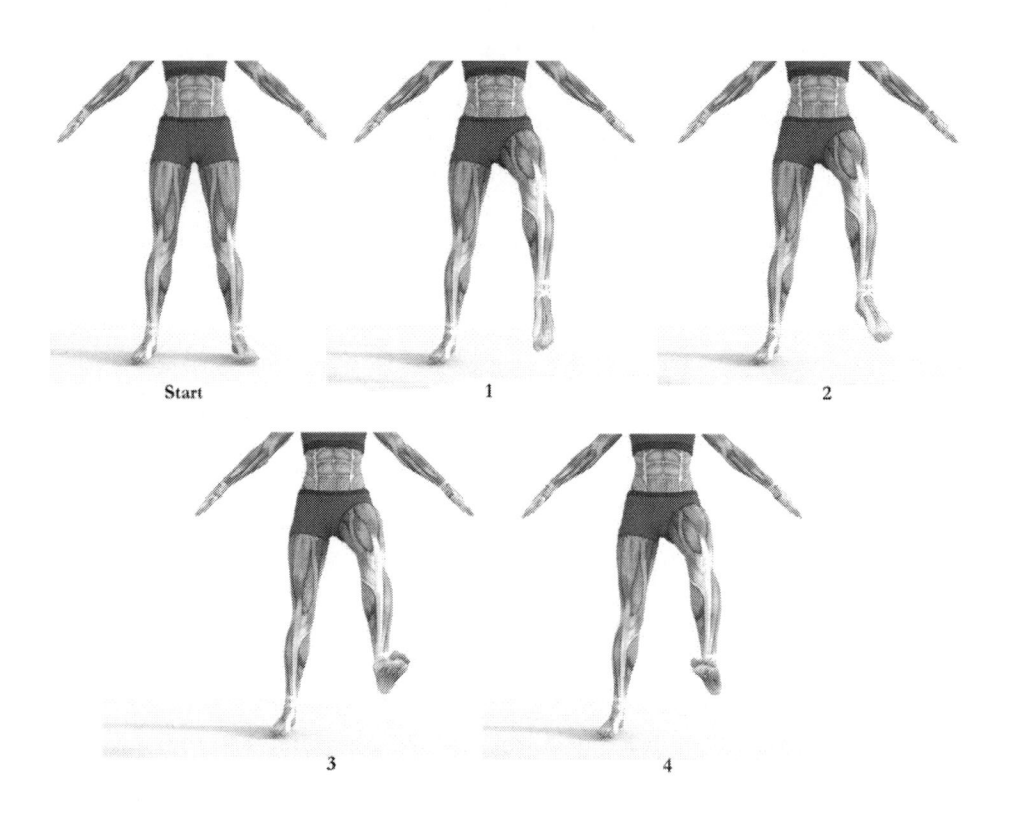

Start position

- This exercises works the ankle joint through its full range of movement
- Keep your back flat, abdominals engaged
- Lift one leg off the floor slightly by bending at the hip and knee and lock this position

Movement

- Drop your foot forward so your toes are pointed towards the floor (1)
- With your toes still pointed down, twist your ankle to the left (2)
- With your toes pointed down and ankle to the left, move your ankle so your toes are pointing upwards (3)
- With your toes pointed up, move your ankle to the right (4)

- From (4) move your ankle so your toes are pointing down and return to the start position. This completes one rotation.

Extra info

You can perform this exercise from a standing or seated position. A good way to look at this exercise is to imagine that you are drawing a circle in the air with your toes. Remember to keep your hip and knee bend as it was in the start position throughout the exercise. Once you have completed your planned amount of rotations on one ankle, switch ankles and repeat.

Waist twist

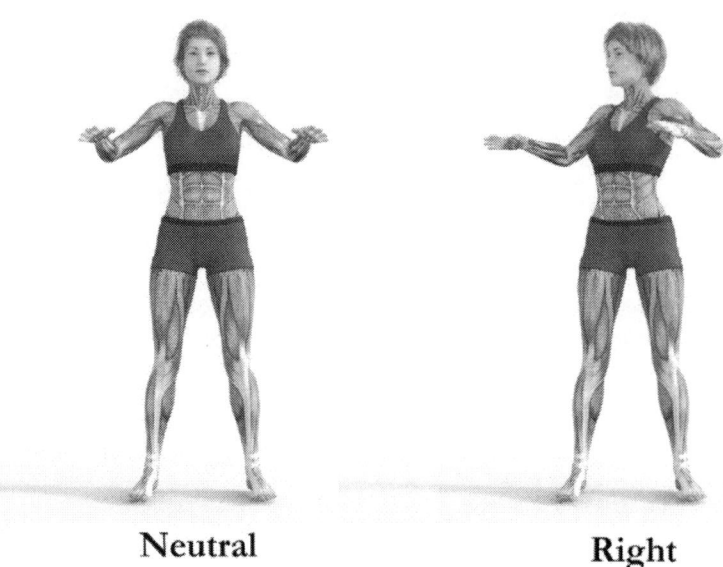

Neutral

Right

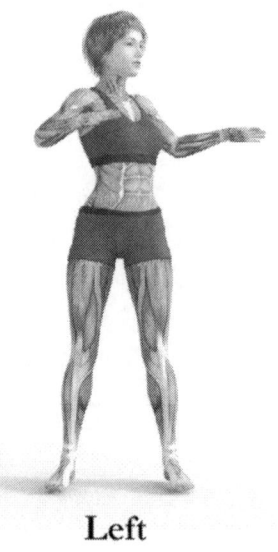

Left

Start position

- This is a range of movement exercise for the abdominals and lower back
- Stand with your knees slightly bent
- Keep your back flat and hips tilted slightly upwards to stabilise your lower back
- Ensure you keep your hips and legs facing forward throughout the exercise

Movement

- From the neutral position, slowly rotate your upper body to the right. Turn your head in this direction also.
- Once at your maximum range of movement to the right, return to the start position and repeat the movement to the left

Extra info

When performing this exercise, you can either stand with your feet together or, as per the diagram, if balance is a problem. Waist twists can be performed whilst in a seated position, but your back should not make contact with the backrest of the chair.

Whether you are performing this exercise from a seated or standing position, your feet should always maintain full contact with the floor and you should always return to the neutral position for a brief pause before starting the movement on the opposite side.

Hip rotation

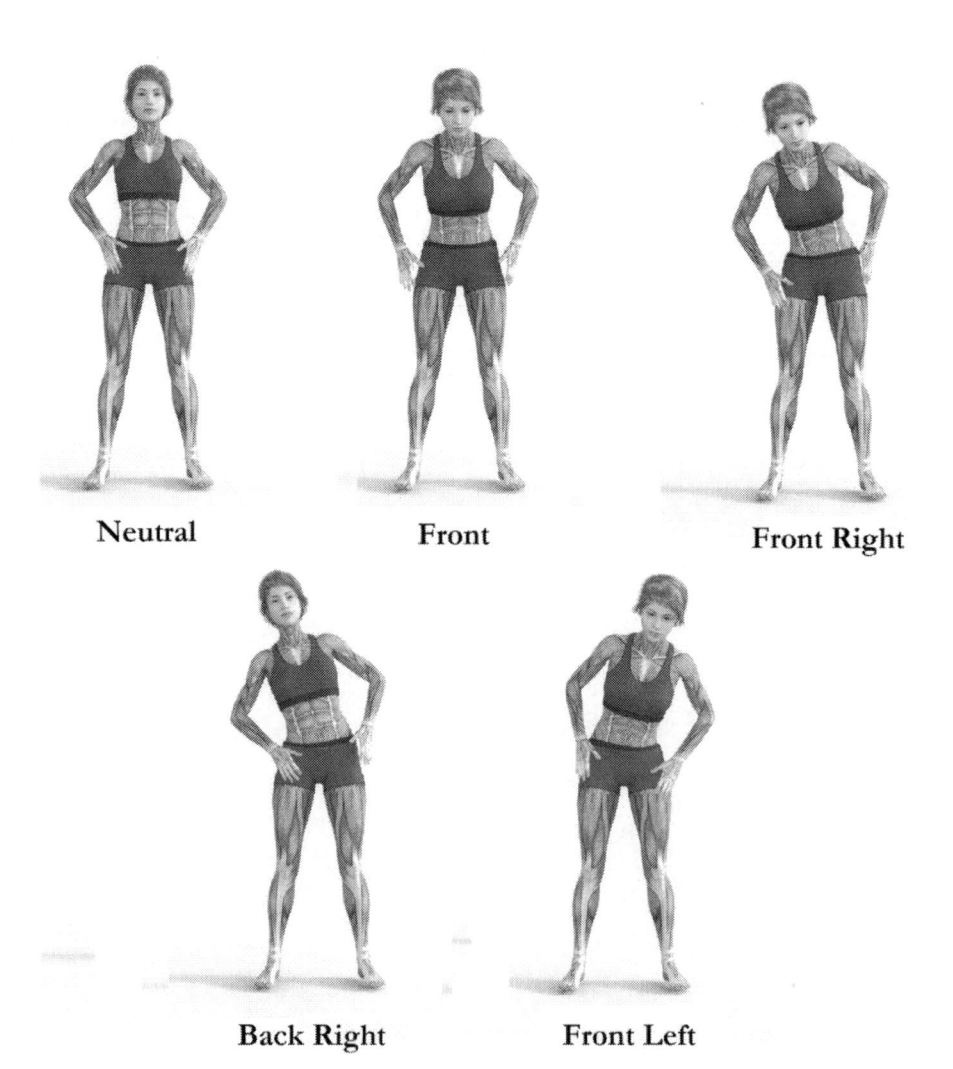

Neutral   Front   Front Right

Back Right   Front Left

Start position

- This is a range of movement exercises for the hips, lower back and abdominals
- Stand with your knees slightly bent and hands on your hips or out in front of you
- Ensure you keep your hips and legs facing forward throughout the exercise

Movement

- From the neutral position, lean your upper body forward slightly hinging at the hips (Front)
- From the front position continue the movement to the right (Front right)
- From the front right position, continue the movement to the back (Back right)
- From the back right, continue the circular movement of the hip rotation back to the front left before returning to the neutral position.

Extra info

This is a continuous, flowing, circular movement of the hips that may take some practice to fully appreciate. Like the ankle rotation exercises, a good way to look at this is to imagine that your head is drawing a circle in the air, but this is all done without moving the lower body.

This exercise should be performed in both directions with full rotations.

Spinal roll down

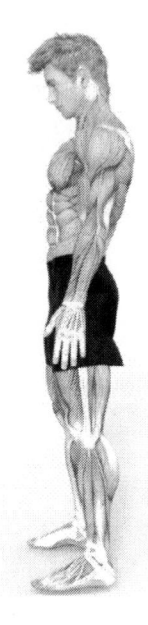

Start

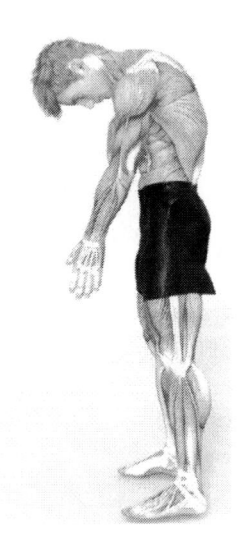

1

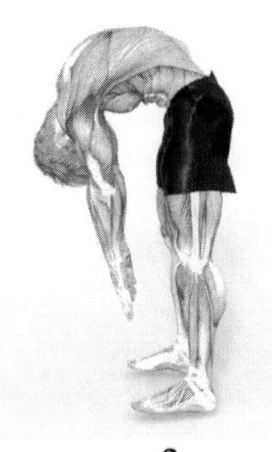

2

Start position

- This is a flexibility exercise for the spine, but it will work the full posterior chain
- Stand up straight with your back flat, knees slightly bent and arms by your sides

Movement

- As you exhale, tuck your chin into your neck whilst bringing your arms to the front and towards your midline
- This will start the roll down of the section of your spine below your neck
- Continue the roll down by pulling your abdominals inwards and reaching to the floor
- Continue further until you are hinging at the hips

Extra info

The range of movement on this exercise will vary drastically from person to person, so if you struggle with it but want to use it in your workouts, just perform the roll down to the point where you are comfortable and work on it incrementally each session.

One thing to be aware of on this exercise is that as your chin is tucked and you are leaning forward, balance may become an issue, it's easy to lose focus and feel yourself falling forward, so have this in mind. A good substitute for this exercises is the "cat cow" if you are too uncomfortable with this one.

Chest opening

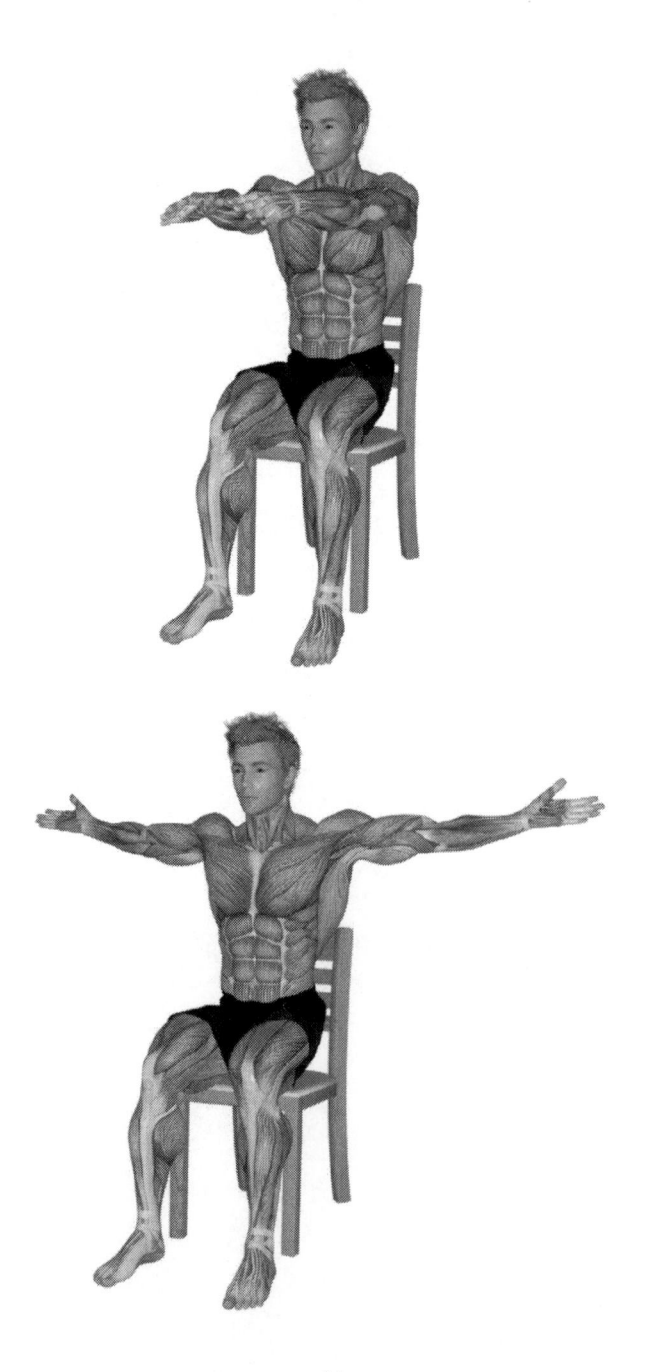

Start position

- This is a range of movement exercises for the chest, but it also offers bicep and rear deltoid movement.
- Sit on a chair with your back flat and not in contact with the back rest
- Your abdominals should be engaged and your arms out in front of you, parallel to the floor, palms facing down and elbows slightly bent
- Your head should be in a neutral position

Movement

- From the start position, as you bring your arms backwards, you should slowly rotate your palms
- Continue the movement until you feel a stretch across your chest
- Your arms should remain parallel to the floor throughout the movement

Extra info

The goal here is to reach the top of movement with your palms facing directly up and your arms directly out to your sides whilst still being parallel to the floor. This exercise looks simple, but it can be a tricky one as there is more going on than a "chest stretch". Bicep and forearm flexors are being challenged here too, so be aware not to perform this movement too quickly. If your elbows want to bend or your palms don't want to rotate, just hold the position you can get to and work on it over time.

Common mistakes are bending the elbows, dropping the arms and rounding the back. So be aware of these, make a mental note of your progress, and don't push too hard.

Shoulder rotation

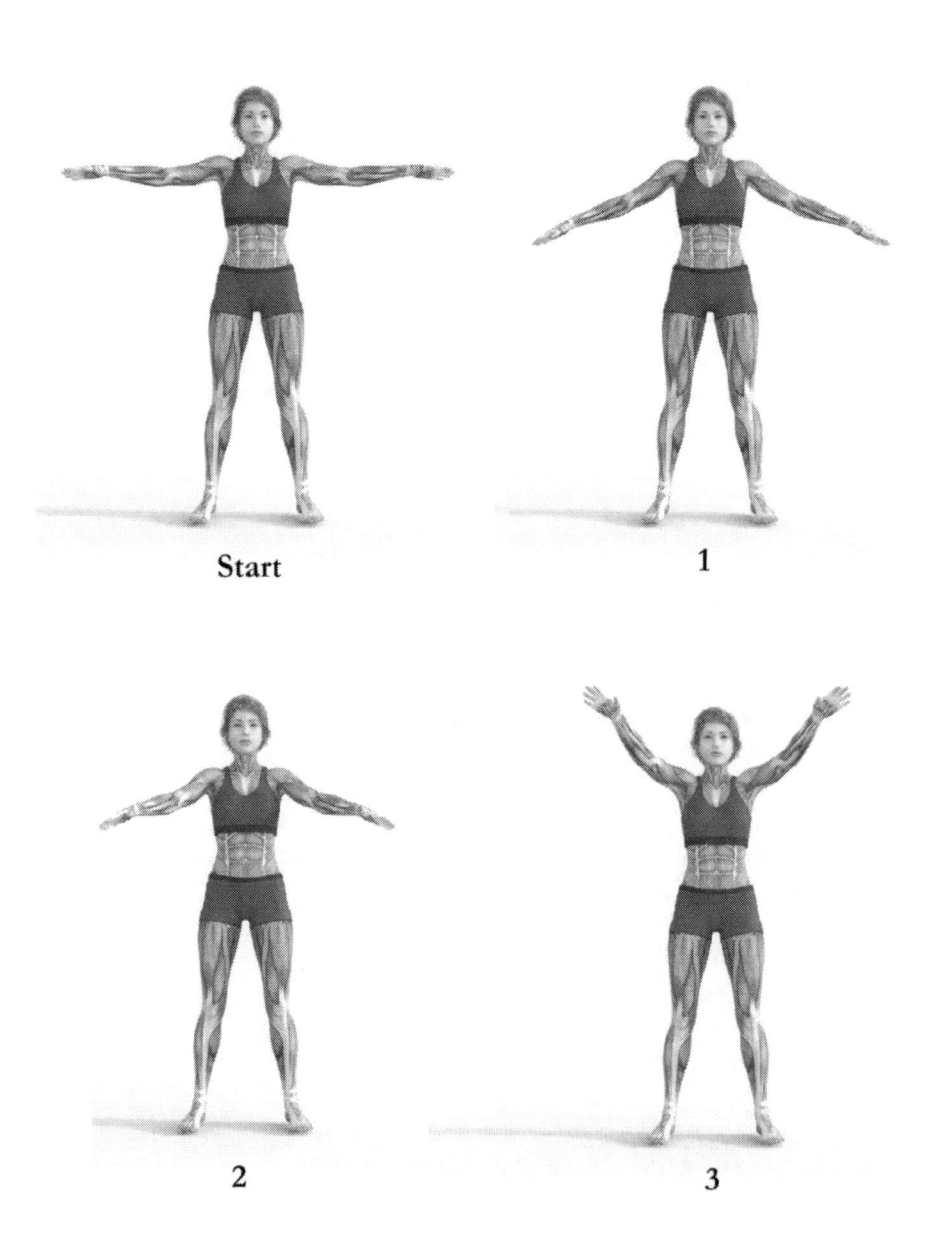

Start

1

2

3

Start position

- This is a range of movement exercises for shoulder rotation and can be used is shoulder strengthening workouts
- Stand or sit so that you have a straight back and engaged abdominals
- Raise your arms directly out to your sides, palms down so they are parallel with the floor (Start)

Movement

- From the start position, keeping your arms straight, lower them towards your sides slightly (1)
- From this position, move your arms forward slightly (2)
- From this position, move your arms up so your hands are higher than your head (3)
- Continue the rotation to bring your arms backwards before returning to position (1). This will complete a full rotation

Extra info

Shoulder rotation can be challenging as we are working against gravity with the weight of our arms. As it is a rotation, the movement will call upon each head of the deltoid to carry this resistance, so it can get tiring fairly quickly.

As with the other rotation exercises, this is a slow, fluid movement and we are drawing small circles in the air with our hands. To make this more challenging and give a better rotation, we can use smaller circular movements or bigger ones. Remember to take is slowly and switch up the direction of rotation evenly in your workouts.

Head & neck mobility

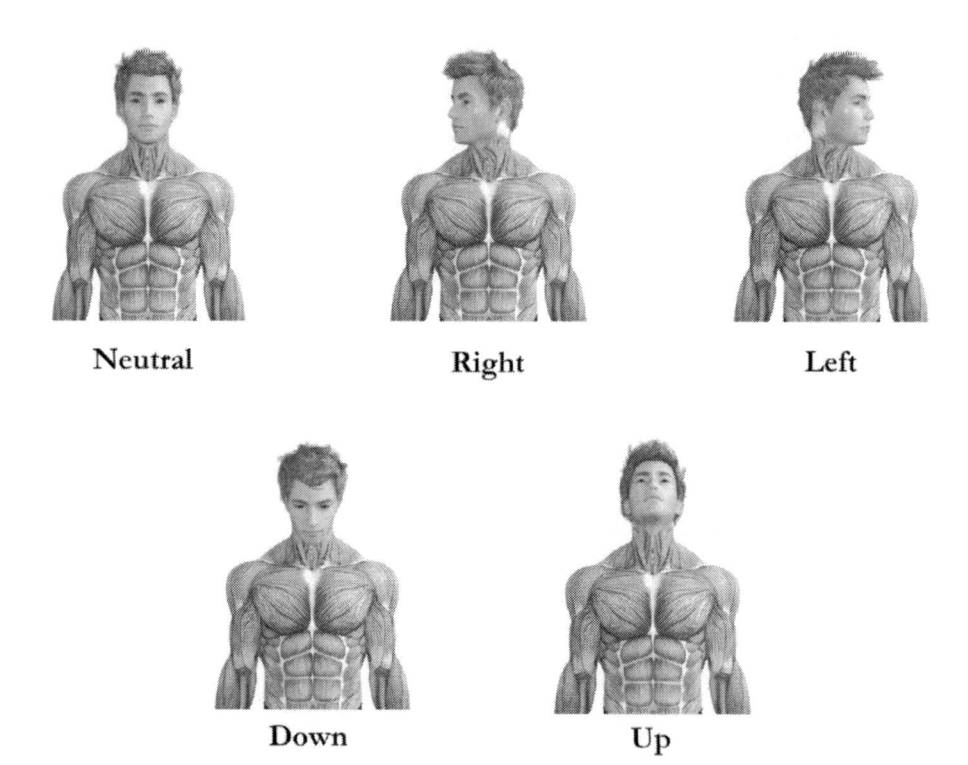

Neutral　　　　Right　　　　Left

Down　　　　Up

Start position

- This is a range of movement exercise for the neck and upper spine
- Sit or stand so that your abs are engaged and your back is flat
- Have your arms relaxed by your sides or in your lap
- Your head should be in a neutral position

Movement

- From the neutral position, keep your torso facing forward and slowly turn your head to the right
- Return to the neutral position before turning your head to the left

- Return to the neutral position before lifting your chin and looking up
- Return to the neutral position before looking down and tucking your chin

Extra info

Unlike other "rotational exercises", these movements all end with a return to the neutral position and a pause before a direction change. I believe this is a safer way to train the neck for mobility as it is not intended to work like a "ball and socket joint".

Although the description takes us through a single directional movement before moving to another, you can hit the same movement multiple times before returning to the neutral position and doing the same for a different direction. For example, you could perform several "up" movements with a return to the neutral position before doing several "down" movements, etc.

However, you do it, these movements should be slow and controlled always.

Spinal extension, flexion – "Cat cow"

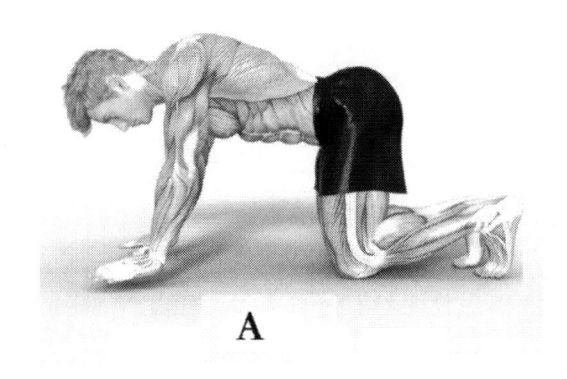

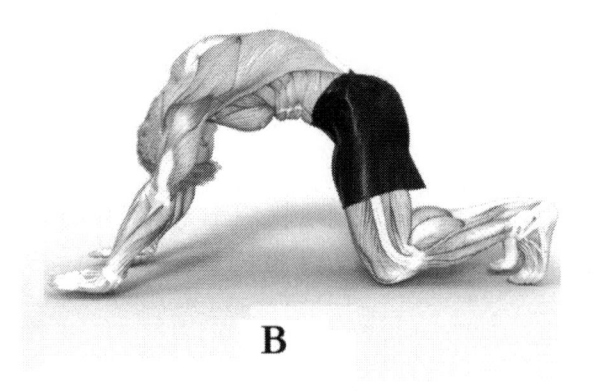

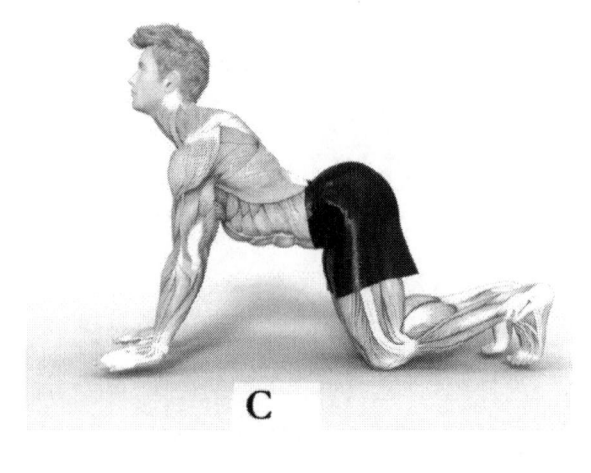

A

B

C

Start position

- This is a mobility exercises for the back
- Take an "all fours position" so that your back is flat, hands, knees and toes are in contact with the floor
- Keep your elbows slightly bent and head in a neutral position

Movement

- From the start position (A), slowly and under control. tuck your chin and move your head forward whilst arching your back upwards and pushing your hips forward (B)
- Hold position (B) for a few seconds
- From position (B), slowly and under control return to the start position (A) and hold for a few seconds
- From position (A), slowly and under control, lift your head so you are looking up and tilt your hips backwards to create slight hyperextension in your lower back

Extra info

This exercise can be used as a substitute for the "spinal roll down". The cat cow does, however, doesn't offer as much potential for challenge as the roll down for the full posterior chain but it offers more stability and also works the spine through hyperextension (when hips are tilted backwards, position "C".

Lower back pain is a common complaint, and this exercise is frequently advised by physiotherapists as a solution for variations of this condition. As it is with every exercise, you should always perform this exercise in a slow and controlled manner and never over extend if you feel uncomfortable.

Seated Exercises

Calf raise seated

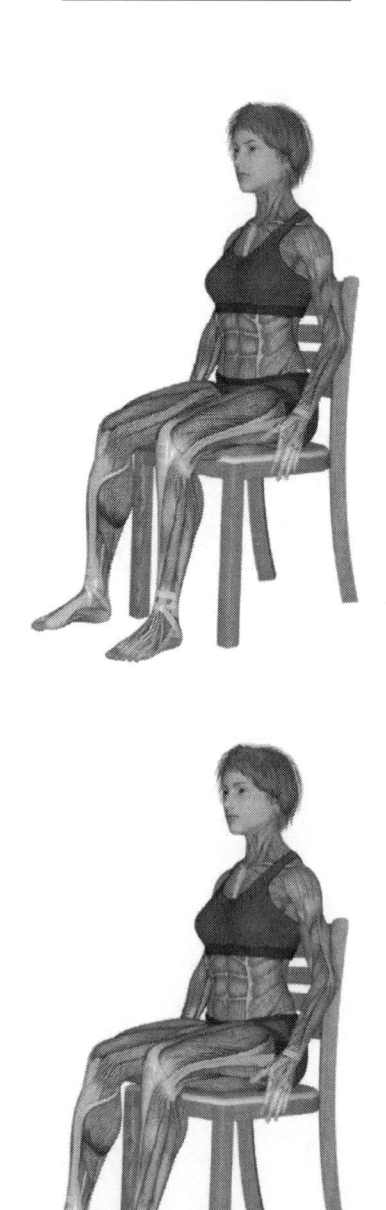

Start position

- This is an exercise to target the calf muscles
- Sit on a chair so your feet are flat to the floor and pointing forwards, keep your back flat, head in a neutral position and abs engaged

Movement

- Keep your toes planted to the floor and as you exhale, bend your ankles so your heels are lifted
- Continue to bend your ankles until you reach full range of motion
- Once at the top of the movement, as you inhale, lower back to the start position

Extra info

You should feel this in your calf muscles (lower, rear legs). It can be fairly intense, so if you are new to this exercise, experiment with the range of movement. As we are all different shapes and sizes, and we will not be working from a standard sized chair, you may also want to experiment with foot positioning. Ideally, you would sit on a chair with your feet flat to the floor and have a right-angle bend in your knees. If you can't get this, try moving your feet towards the chair or further away. You can even bring them close together or further apart. But they should always face directly forward.

Seated Low row

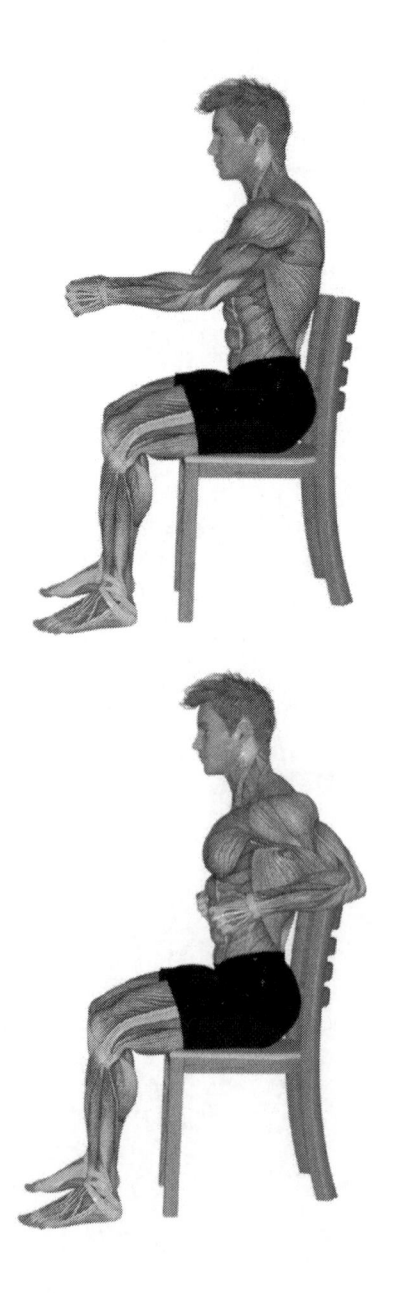

Start position

- This is an exercise that targets the back muscles
- Sit on a chair so your feet are flat to the floor and pointing forwards, keep your back flat, head in a neutral position and abs engaged
- Lift your lower arms so they are parallel with the floor and push your shoulders forward
- Push your upper arms forward slightly so they are at about a 45 degree angle to your torso

Movement

- As you exhale, pull your shoulders back and push your chest forward
- Continue pulling your elbows back so they end up behind your torso
- Your hands should end up in line with your lower abdominals
- Once at the top of movement, as you inhale, return to the start position

Extra info

Rows are an excellent exercise for working the back muscles, including the rear deltoids and traps. Many people struggle to connect with back muscles, including myself when I was a beginner. This very exercise helped me to understand the function of my latissimus dorsi and help me build this muscle group up to bodybuilding competition standard.

The back muscles are a big group and handle a lot of movements, so this can be a valuable exercise. During the exercise, it's important not to arch your back or drop your head.

Seated hip hinge

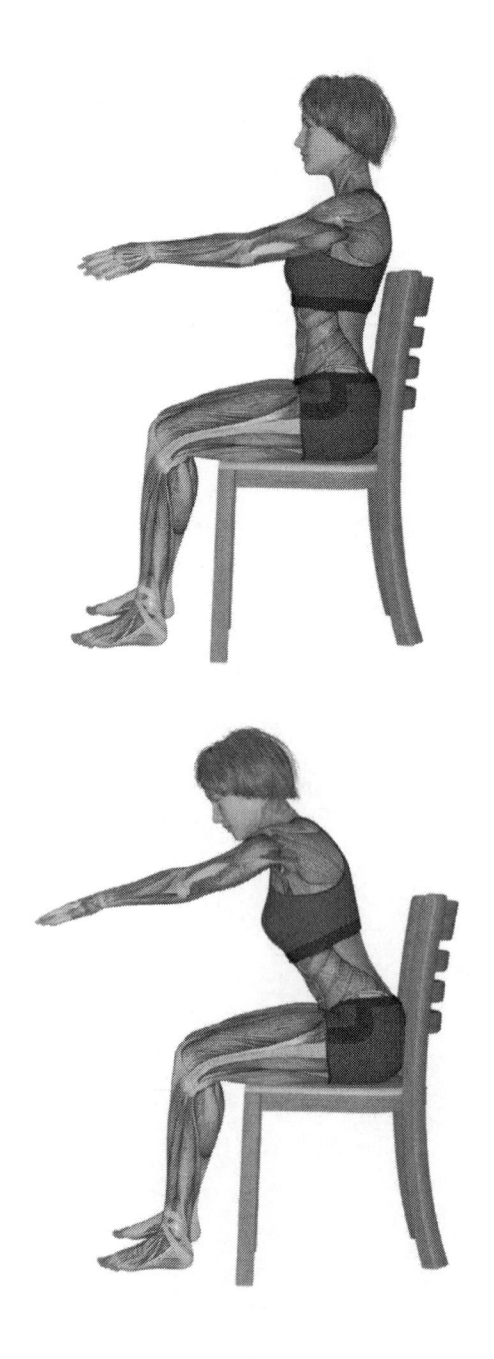

Start position

- This is an exercise to target the lower back, but it also has engagement of the abs and glutes
- Sit on a chair so your feet are flat to the floor and pointing forwards, keep your back flat and head in a neutral position
- Engage your glutes and abdominals
- Lift your arms so they are out to your front and about parallel to the floor

Movement

- As you exhale, hinge at the hips so that your torso moves forward
- Your feet should remain in full contact with the floor
- Continue hinging at the hips until you feel a stretch in your lower back
- Once at the top of movement, as you inhale, return to the start position

Extra info

Keeping your glutes and abdominals engaged on this one is important. Not only will it help to control the movement, but it will help to support your lower back and strengthen these muscle groups, too.

Shoulder reach

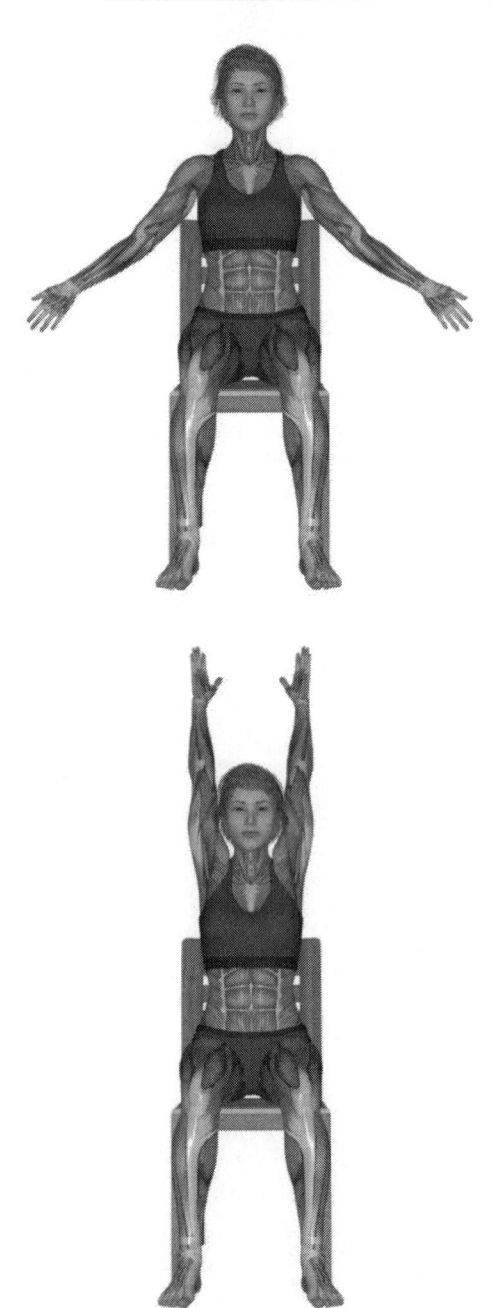

Start position

- This is an a hybrid exercise that develops range of movement of the shoulder joint whist also challenges the deltoid muscles
- Sit on a chair so your feet are flat to the floor and pointing forwards, keep your back flat and head in a neutral position
- Engage your glutes and abdominals for stability
- Set your arms so they are straight with a slight bend at the elbows and palms facing forward

Movement

- As you exhale, lift your arms upwards by bending the shoulder joint
- As you raise your arms, rotate your palms so they are facing towards your body's mid line
- Keep your arms straight and aim to finish with your hands directly above your head
- Once at the top of movement, hold for a few seconds and return to the start position as you inhale

Extra info

This movement can be challenging at first, but it's also one that can be worked on regularly. Bending at the elbows will make it easier to progress to complete the movement, but it will also dilute the exercise. The top of movement can be pushed further by having your palms touch directly above your head with your arms straight.

Knee bend

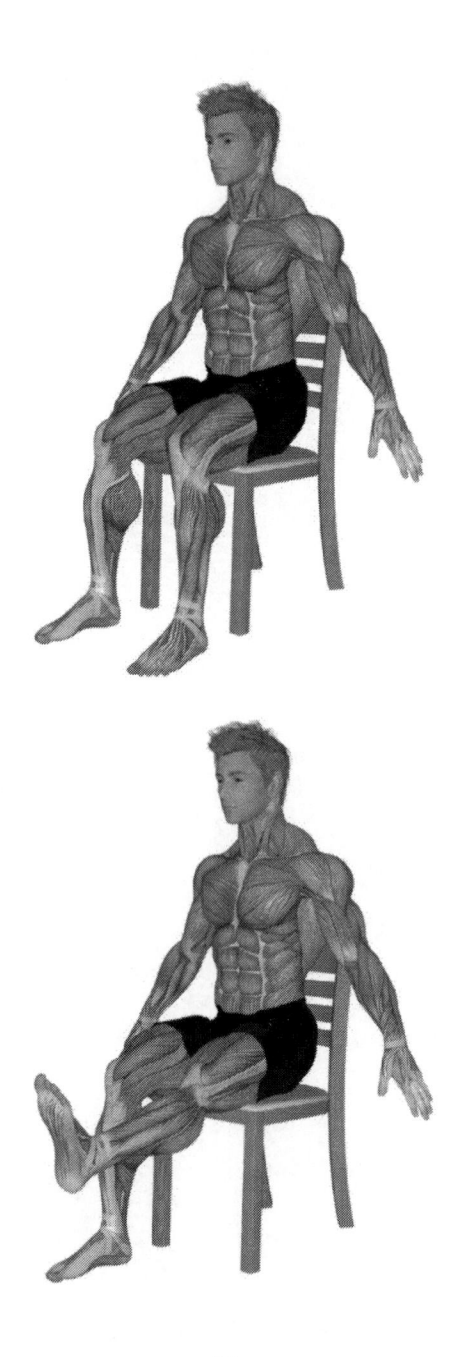

Start position

- This is a single muscle exercise to target the quad muscles (upper front leg).
- Sit on a chair so that your back is flat, head is in the neutral position and feet are flat on the floor
- Feet should be about hip width apart

Movement

- Engage your abs and glutes
- As you exhale, raise one of your lower legs by bending at the knee until it is just about to lock out
- Keep your toes pointed upwards
- Once at the top of movement, as you inhale, return to the start position
- Repeat for your planned amount of reps and then repeat on the opposite leg

Extra info

Although this is an isolation exercise for the quads, it requires other stabiliser muscles to be engaged. Tight hamstrings may also cause a lack of range of movement, but having our toes pointed, (maintaining a right angle between the shin and the top of the foot) will help to develop flexibility in the hamstrings.

Beginners to this exercise may find it useful for stability if they hold on to the side of the chair for extra support. This can also make the exercise more effective for the quads if stability is an issue.

Leg lift - knee bent

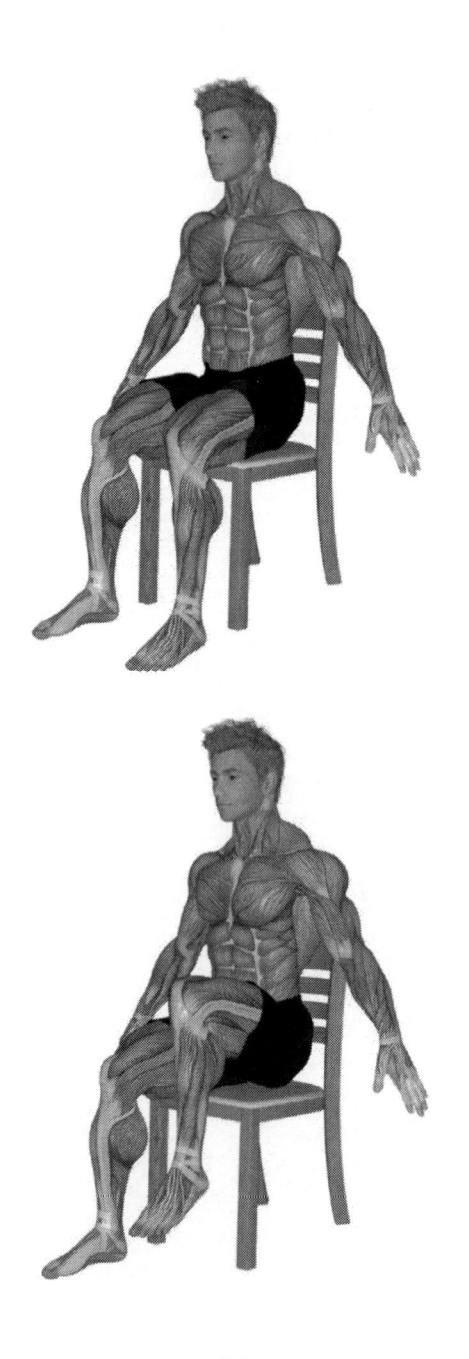

Start position

- This is an exercise to target the quad muscles and hip flexors
- Sit on a chair so that your back is flat, head is in the neutral position and feet are flat on the floor
- Feet should be about hip width apart

Movement

- As you exhale, lift one of your legs up by flexing at the hip
- The bend in your knee should not change throughout the movement
- Your torso should also remain as per the start position
- Once you are at the top of movement, hold for a few seconds and return to the start position as you inhale

Extra info

As this is a similar exercise to the knee bend, it can be beneficial for beginners to hold on to the side of the chair for extra stability.

Leg widening

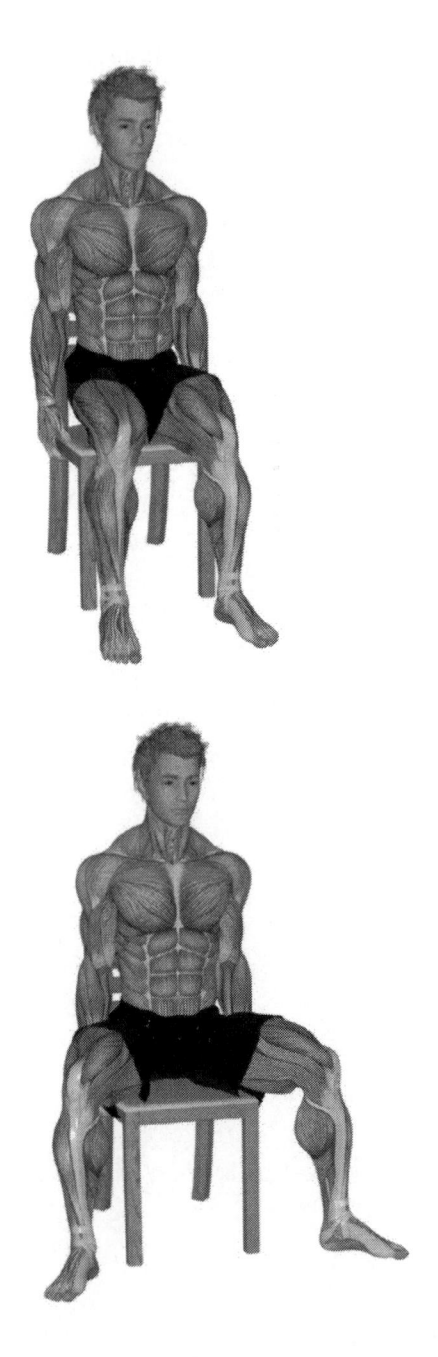

Start position

- This is an exercise to target the adductors, abductors and hip flexors
- Sit on a chair so that your back is flat, head is in the neutral position and feet are flat on the floor
- Feet should be about hip width apart
- Hold onto the sides of the chair for stability

Movement

- As you exhale, make sure your abs and glutes are engaged before you lift both feet so they are slightly off the floor
- Move your legs away from your midline to widen your stance
- Once at the top of movement, hold for a few seconds before inhaling and returning to the start position

Extra info

Although it is possible to do this exercise without support, I'd advise that it is performed by holding onto the chair. The slight "knees up action" may put undue pressure on the lower back. Regarding the movement, you can either keep your feet off the floor through the entire set or you can place them back on the floor between reps. Keeping your feet off the floor through the entire set will increase strength in the hip flexors, but this can be challenging for some, dependent on the rep range.

Seated waist twist

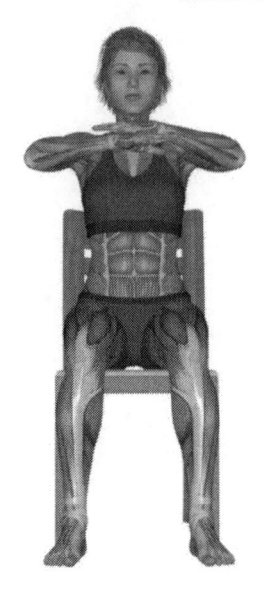

Neutral

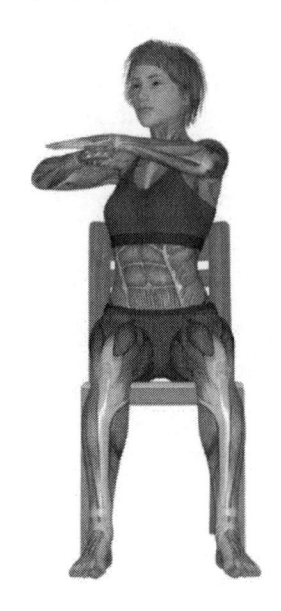

Right

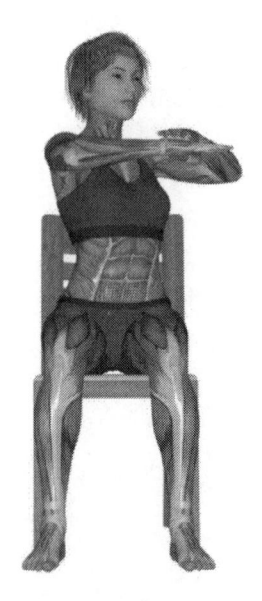

Left

Start position

- This is an exercise for lower back and core flexibility
- Sit on a chair so that your back is flat, head is in the neutral position and feet are flat on the floor
- Feet should be about hip width apart
- Raise your arms, cross them so they are out in front of you and parallel to the floor

Movement

- As you exhale, slowly and under control twist at your waist to rotate your upper body to the right
- Once you are at the top of movement, pause and return to the start position (neutral) as you inhale
- After a short pause at the neutral position, repeat the waist twist in the opposite direction

Extra info

This is a great exercise for mobility through the lower back and core, but it must be performed under control and I advised that a short pause at the neutral position before rotating in the opposite direction is always used. This is to help with a "start position reset" and to stop any chance of momentum.

Single movement exercises

Hover sit

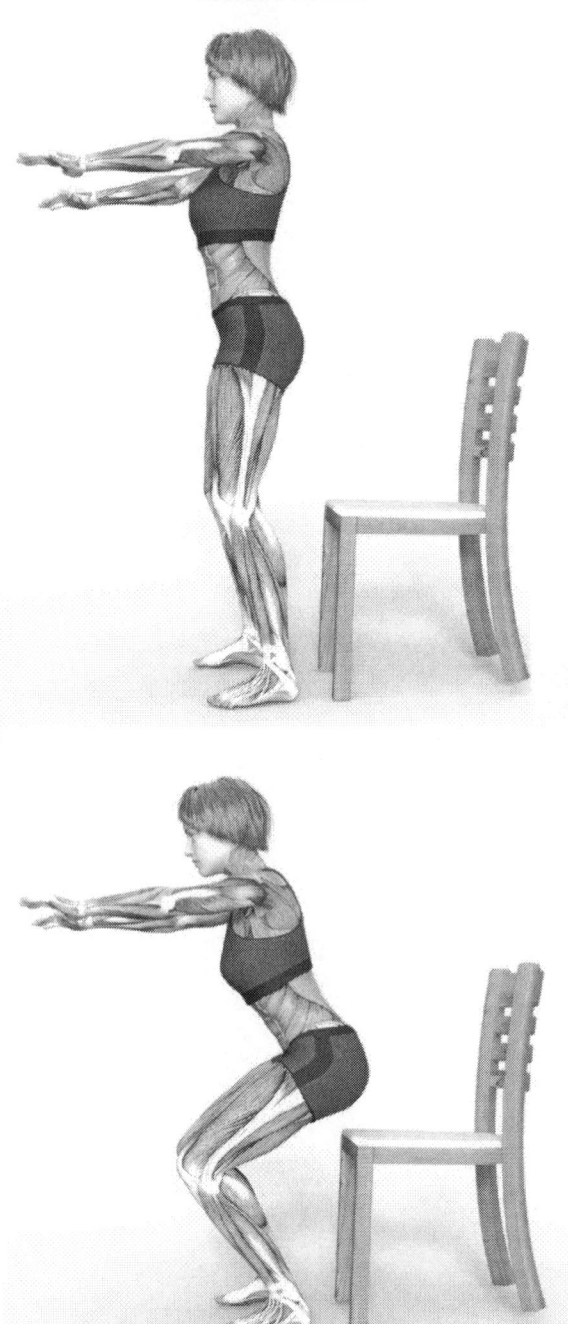

Start position

- This is an exercise to target the quads and glutes
- Stand in front of a chair as if you were about to sit on it
- Keep your back flat, head in the neutral position and feet about shoulder width apart
- Raise your arms so they are parallel to the floor and out in front of you

Movement

- As you inhale, bend at the knees to lower your bum towards the chair
- Ensure that your knees continue to point forwards or slightly out to the sides
- Your back should remain flat and arms parallel to the floor
- Lower yourself until your glutes graze the seat on the chair
- Once you reach the top of movement, exhale and return to the start position

Extra info

This is, in effect, a progression to a full bodyweight squat. Many trainers new to squats have weaker glutes, which gives a lack of confidence to practise squatting movements. The chair in this exercise makes for a great safety barrier to boost this confidence.

When practicing this exercise, it is possible to actually touch the chair with your glutes, as long as you don't take the weight of your body off your glutes and legs, this is a great way to develop a deeper squat, until you no longer need the chair.

Single leg balance

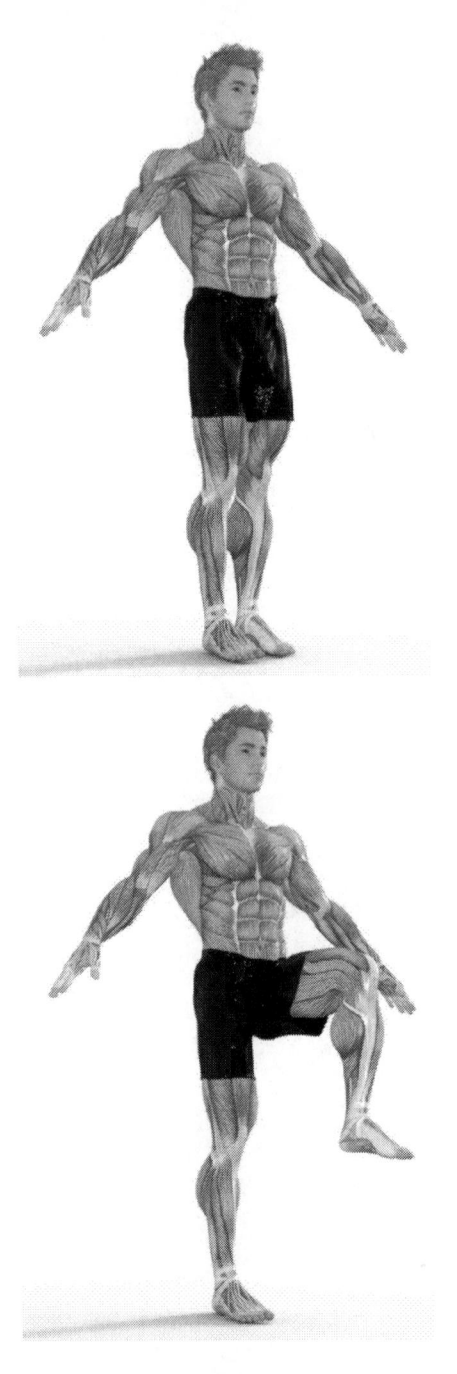

Start position

- This is an exercise that develops stabiliser muscles not only in the legs, but throughout the body
- Stand with your feet and knees together, back flat and arms out to the sides for stability
- Knees should have a slight bend in them so they are not locked out

Movement

- As you exhale, lift one leg by bending at the hip and knee
- Your back should be flat and supporting foot should be planted on the floor
- Once at the top of movement, hold for the planned amount of time before returning to the start position
- Repeat the process on the opposite leg

Extra info

As this exercise is a test of balance, I would advise that you plan a time to hold at the top of movement based on your ability. This can be increased as you become stronger.

The range of movement is something else to work on. Ideally, the top of movement should be as the illustration shows, where the upper leg is lifted, so it is parallel to the floor, but this can also be something to work on. If you are new to this exercise, lifting your leg slightly off the floor is a good starting point and a bigger range of movement and longer time holding the position can be future progressions.

Bicep curl

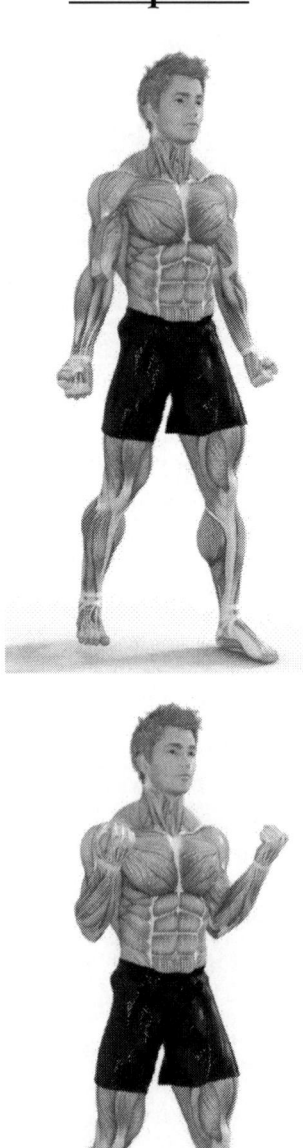

Start position

- This is an exercise to target the biceps
- Stand with one foot in front of the other for stability
- Engage your abdominals, keep your back flat and head in a neutral position
- Straighten your arms so they are by your sides and have your palms facing forward before making fists with your hands
- Roll your shoulders back so your biceps are facing forwards

Movement

- As you exhale, bend at the elbows to bring your fists towards your biceps
- Keep your back flat and shoulders rolled back during the exercise
- Once at the top of movement, as you inhale, return to the start position

Extra info

This exercise is a classic way to target the bicep muscles. The stance can be as described in the description, or it can be with your feet and knees together. The idea of the "one foot in front of the other" stance is to create stability if you decide to perform this exercise with a barbell or dumbbells in the future.

Tricep extension

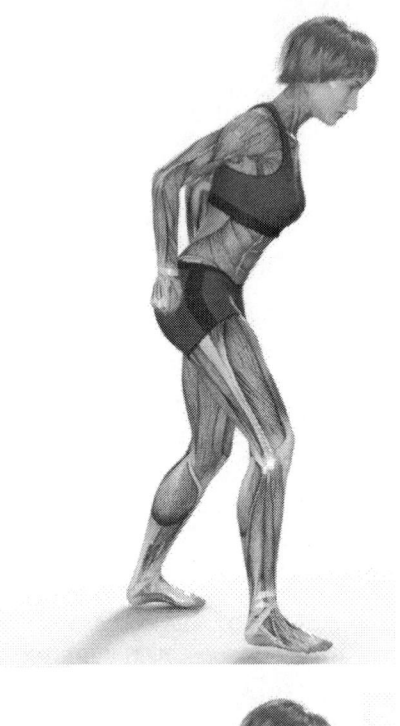

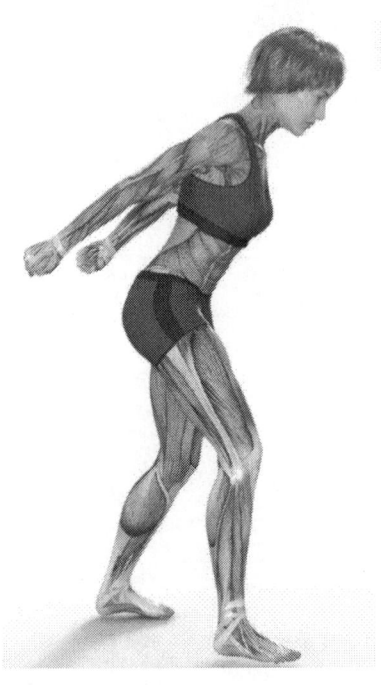

Start position

- This is an exercise to target the triceps
- Stand with one foot in front of the other for stability
- Engage your abdominals, keep your back flat and head in a neutral position
- Hinge forward slightly at the hips but maintain a flat back
- Lift your upper arms slightly so your elbows are higher than your back line
- Your elbows should also be bent

Movement

- As you exhale, whilst maintaining the position of your upper arms, straighten your lower arms by bending at the elbows
- Once at the top of movement, as you inhale, return to the start position

Extra info

Although this exercise looks simple, tricep extensions can be tricky to get right. Remember to keep your upper arms high and fixed throughout the movement as it's easy to allow them to lower without noticing. This will dilute the workload to the triceps.

Hip extension

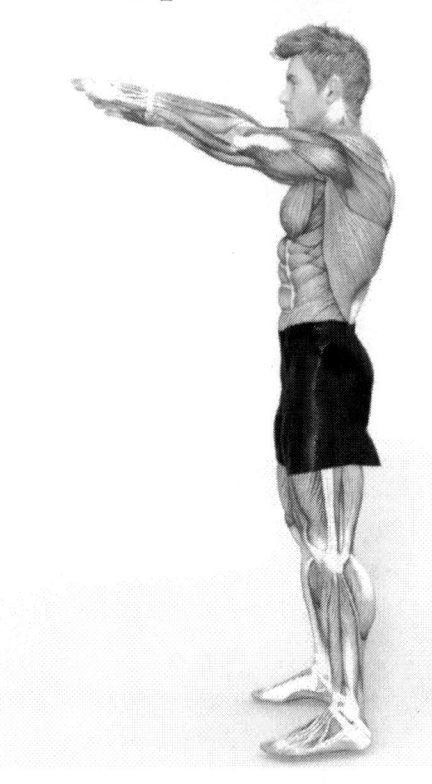

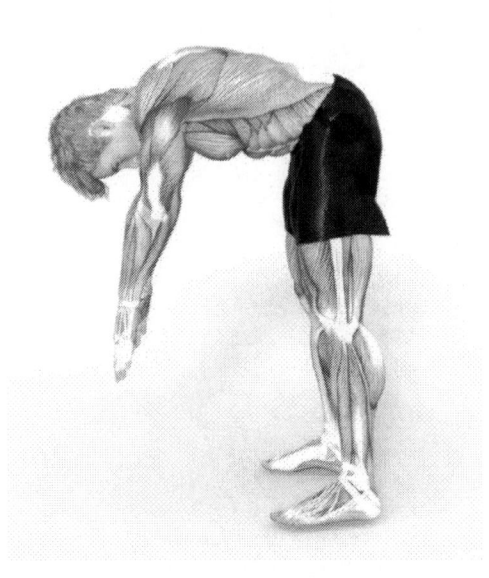

Start position

- This is an exercise to improve flexibility through the hips and hamstrings and to strengthen the lower back
- Stand with your back flat, head in a neutral position and feet about hip width apart
- Raise your arms out in front of you so they are parallel with the floor

Movement

- As you exhale, slowly and under control, hinge at the hips to lower your upper body towards the floor
- Keep a slight bend in your knees, but your legs should be straight
- Once your torso is about parallel to the floor, slowly tuck your chin towards your chest
- Once at the top of movement, slowly and under control, return to the start position
-

Extra info

Hip extension is a great exercise for flexibility. The closer to the floor your fingers can reach, the more progressed you are with the exercise. If you can touch your toes without bending your knees, you are doing very well!

Seated crunch

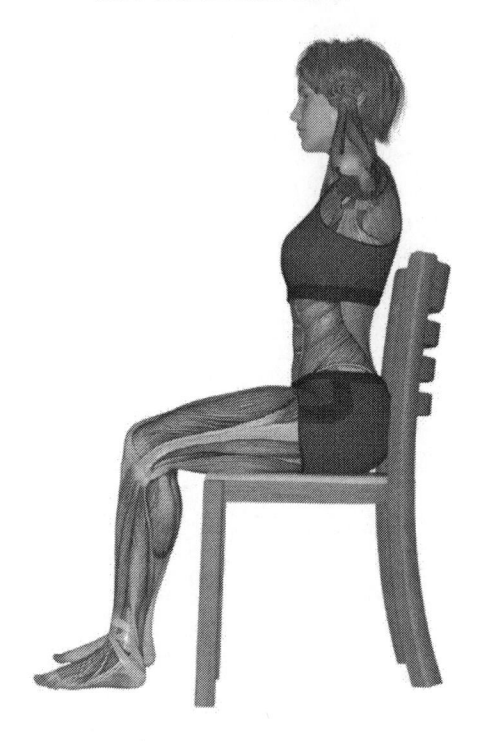

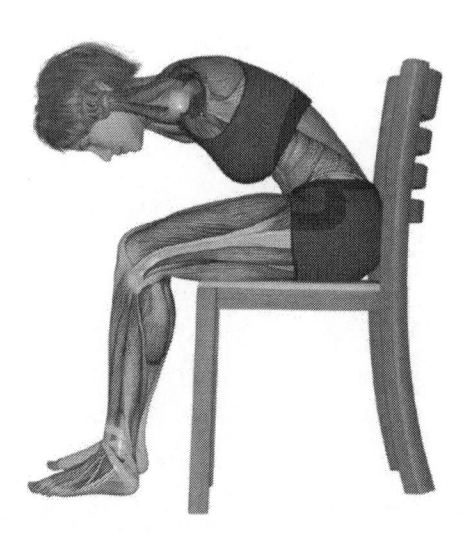

Start position

- This is an exercise to target the abdominals
- Sit on a chair so your feet are flat to the floor, back is flat and head in a neutral position
- Raise your arms and hands so your fingers rest on the sides of your head

Movement

- Before you start the movement, engage your abdominals and glutes
- As you exhale, hinge at the waist to "crunch" in your abdominals. This should cause your mid back to round
- Once you reach the top of movement, as you inhale, return to the start position

Extra info

Crunches and abdominal exercises can be performed in many ways, but this is a basic exercise to familiarise ourselves with the function of the abdominals and form a foundation for crunch and other abdominal exercise progression.

Lateral raises

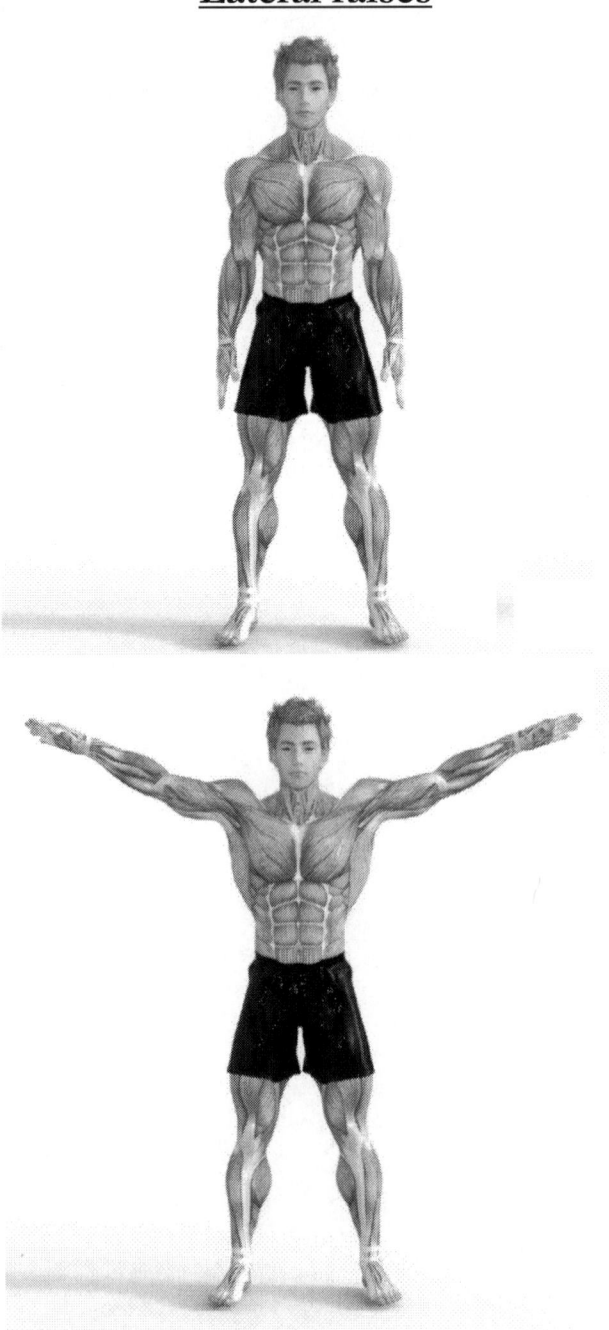

Start position

- This is an exercise to target the mid deltoids (shoulders)
- Stand with your feet about shoulder width apart, back flat and head in a neutral position
- Straighten your arms and have them by your sides, palms facing inwards

Movement

- As you exhale, raise your arms out to your sides keeping them in line with your body
- Continue raising your arms until they are just above parallel with the floor
- Once at the top of movement, return to the start position

Extra info

This is another exercise that may look simple, but it can be tricky for some. A common mistake with lateral raises is to allow the arms to move forward during the movement. This will dilute the workload to the lateral deltoid and allow an often stronger front deltoid to take over. If you use this exercise in your workouts, this is something to look out for.

Front raises

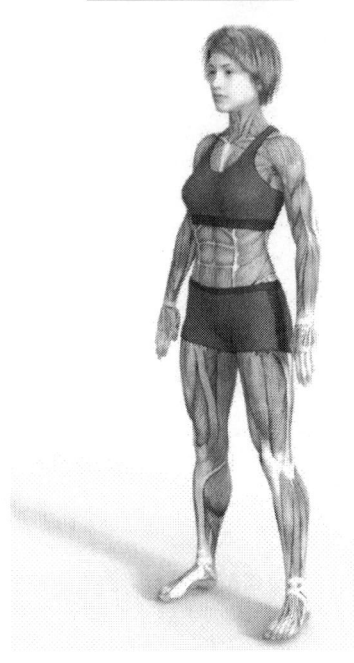

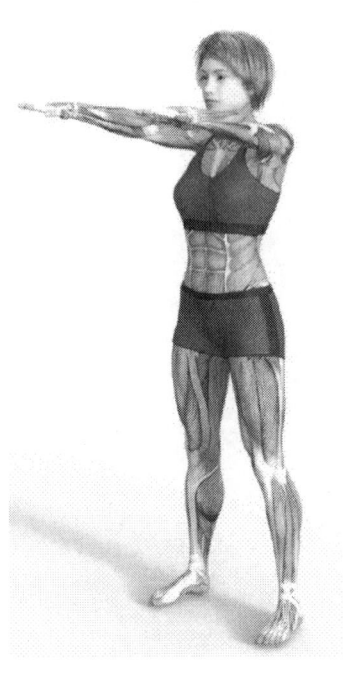

Start position

- This is an exercise to target the front deltoid (shoulder)
- Stand with your feet about shoulder width apart, back flat and head in a neutral position
- Straighten your arms and have them by your sides, palms facing inwards

Movement

- As you exhale, raise your arms out to your front keeping them about shoulder width apart
- As you perform this movement, progressively rotate your palms so the finish facing downwards
- Continue raising your arms until they are just above parallel with the floor
- Once at the top of movement, return to the start position

Extra info

Front deltoids are often stronger muscles than the lateral and rear deltoids, so these may feel easier than the lateral movement. If you are working on shoulder strength and mobility, the two exercises may be a good fit for the same workout.

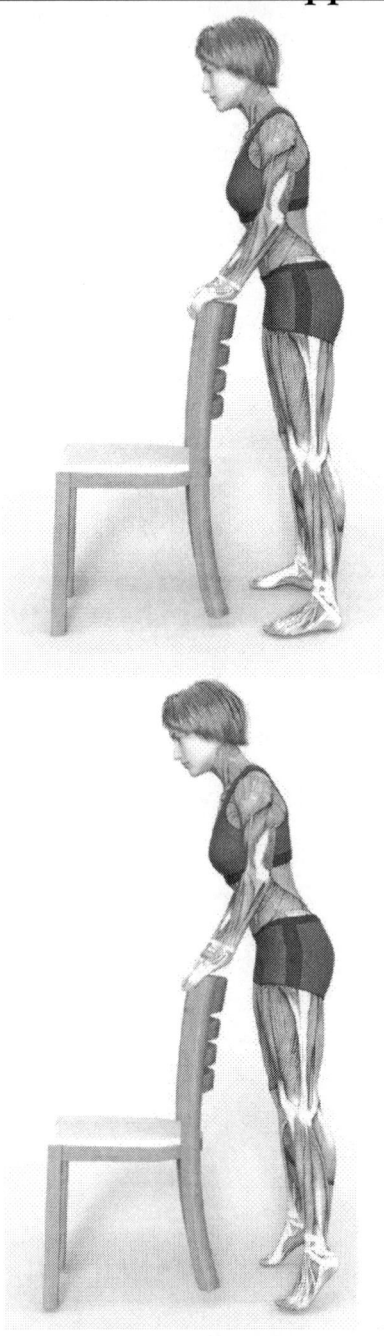

Calf raises with support

Start position

- This is an exercise to target the calf muscles (lower leg)
- Stand behind a high backed chair with your feet spaced about hip width apart
- Use the chair for support by holding onto it, but do not use it to take the weight of your body
- Hinge at the hips slightly if you need to but keep the rest of your back flat
- Keep your legs straight, but have a slight bend in your knees

Movement

- As you exhale, push through the front of your feet to move onto your toes
- Continue this weight transfer until your are fully on your tip toes
- Once at the top of movement, as you inhale, return to the start position

Extra info

Calf raises can be an intense exercise, as the muscles are denser than other muscle groups. Ensure that you make this movement in a slow and controlled manner.

The illustration shows a chair as support, but we can use anything that is solid, such as a wall. It's important to remember that this support is only used for balance, so we should not use it as an aid in weight bearing as this will dilute the exercise benefits.

Side bends

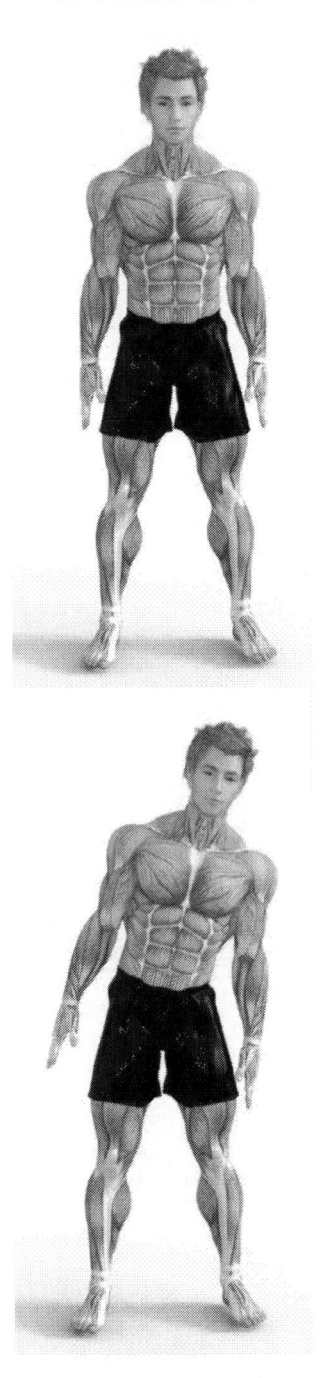

Start position

- This is an exercise to target the side of the abdominals
- Stand with your feet about shoulder width apart, back flat and head in a neutral position
- Straighten your arms and have them by your sides, palms facing inwards

Movement

- As you exhale, bend to one side through your mid abdominal
- Keep your back flat. Your torso should not move backwards or forwards
- Continue the movement by reaching down your outer leg with the hand on the working side.
- Once at the top of the movement, as you exhale, return to the starting position

Extra info

With side bends, it's easy to either lean your upper body forward or backwards when performing the exercise, and this is not what we want. If you are new to this exercise, focus on keeping the correct alignment as a priority before increasing the range of movement.

Dorsal raise

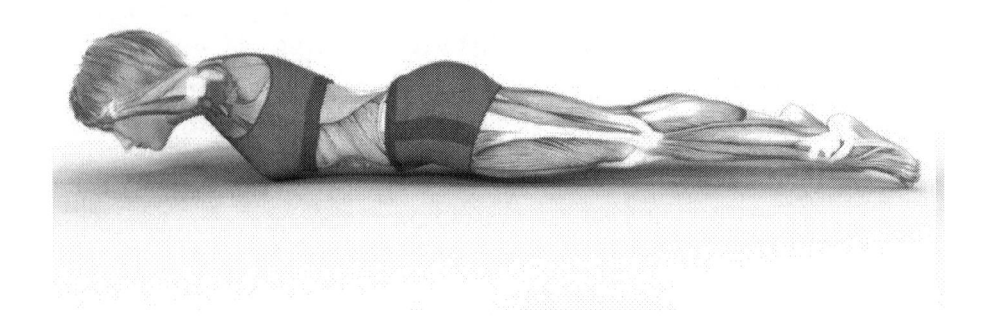

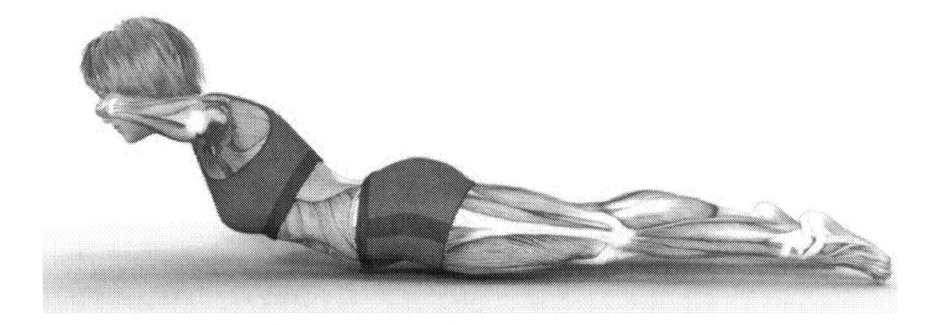

Start position

- This is an exercise to target the lower back
- Lay flat on the floor with your head in the neutral position.
- The tops of your feet should be in contact with the floor and your legs straight.
- Bring your arms up and to your sides, placing your fingers on your temples.
- Engage your core and glutes and lift your head slightly away from the floor.

Movement

- As you exhale, lift your upper body away from the floor.
- Keep your glutes engaged.
- Keep your feet in contact with the floor.

- Keep your arms in the start position.
- Only raise your upper body to where you feel the tension.
- Once at the top of movement, inhale and return to the start position.

Extra info

This is a small movement, and there is an element of back hyper extension. So it's really important to keep this movement slow, controlled and smooth. If this is a new exercise, approach it with caution and test your range of movement abilities.

There is no need to over extend on this, you can benefit from small movements and the engagement alone.

The stabiliser

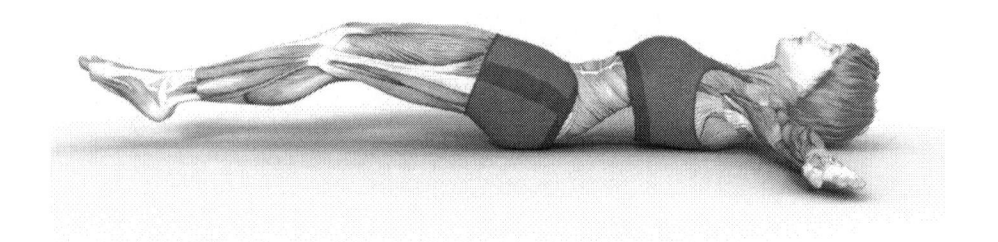

Start position

- This is an isometric exercise to target core strength
- Lay flat on the floor, keeping your legs straight, feet together and flat on the floor.
- Tilt your hips slightly to push your lower back into the floor.
- Engage your abdominals and glutes and lift one foot about an inch off the floor. This will be the "moving leg".
- Place your arms out to your sides, palms down and flat to the floor for stability.
- Ensure that your head and back are in contact with the floor throughout the movement.

Movement

- This is an isometric hold and should be used based on the individual's ability.
- Ensure to maintain glute and abdominal engagement throughout the hold.
- Breathing should be slow and controlled throughout the hold.

Extra info

This exercise engages the lower abs and lower back. To make this effective for lower back stability, focus on keeping your glutes engaged and your lower back pushed into the floor by tilting your hips.

Multi movement exercises

Wall push ups

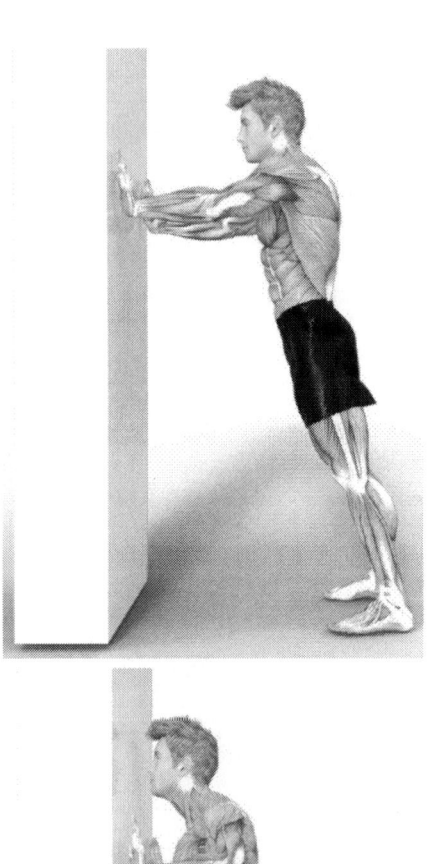

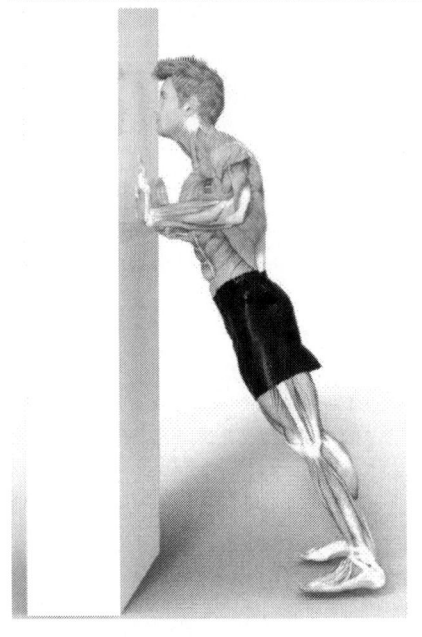

Start position

- This exercise targets the chest and tricep muscles
- Find a solid, upright surface to work with. A straight wall is ideal.
- Position your hands on the wall so your arms are parallel to the floor and in line with your mid chest.
- Make sure your hands are spaced so that your thumbs are in line with your outer shoulder.
- Take a step backwards so that you are taking the weight of your body.
- Keep your back flat, abs engaged and look forward.

Movement

- As you inhale, bend your arms by lowering your body towards the wall until your nose almost touches the surface.
- Your elbows should flare out only slightly.
- Once at the top of the movement, exhale as you return to the start position. This is one rep.

Extra info

Lowering yourself until your nose touches the surface will serve as a good gauge for maximum range of movement and will help you keep your back straight. Remember that the further you step back while setting up your position, the more challenging it will be, but the more of an incline that you create here will put a bigger workload on the shoulders and may take from the chest, so there is a fine line.

Step ups

A

B

C

Start position

- This is an exercise to simulate walking up steps to target the leg muscles
- Find a solid raised surface that will take your weight
- Stand in front of the step so your toes are a few inches away from it (A)

Movement

- As you exhale, step forward with one foot onto the step (B)
- Once the forward foot is planted firmly on the step, follow with the other foot (C)
- With both feet planted firmly onto the step, reverse the process to finish a full "step up"

Extra info

Step ups can work on the muscles that are needed for walking up steps, but they can also be used for cardio sessions. If you decide to use this exercise in your workouts, you can either use them as a times exercise or perform a set amount of reps. If you choose to use the "sets and reps" method, note that a single rep is counted only after reaching the start position again (shown in figure (A).

The higher the step, the more challenging this will be. Remember to focus on keeping a flat back and perform the movement with a slight pause after each step so momentum does not creep in.

Step & reach

A

B

C

Start position

- This is an exercise to simulate walking up steps to target the leg muscles whist also working on shoulder mobility
- Find a solid raised surface that will take your weight
- Stand in front of the step so your toes are a few inches away from it (A)

Movement

- As you step onto the surface, start to lift your arms in front of you
- Your arms should be straight and about shoulder width apart
- Once your leading foot is firmly planted onto the surface, follow with your other foot
- As your trailing foot is planted onto the step, you should continue lifting your arms until they are straight above your head
- Hold this position for a few seconds
- Once at the top of movement, reverse the process

Extra info

This exercise requires a bit more coordination than step ups, so I would advise that you are comfortable with the step ups exercise before moving onto this one. There will also be an added challenge of balance with the step and reach, so this is something to be aware of.

This is another exercise that requires extra concentration to stop momentum taking over the exercise. If you pause at each stage slightly, there will be no momentum and you will get the most out of the movement. With that said, it is still possible with practice to make this movement a fluid one and still get good value from it.

Twist & reach

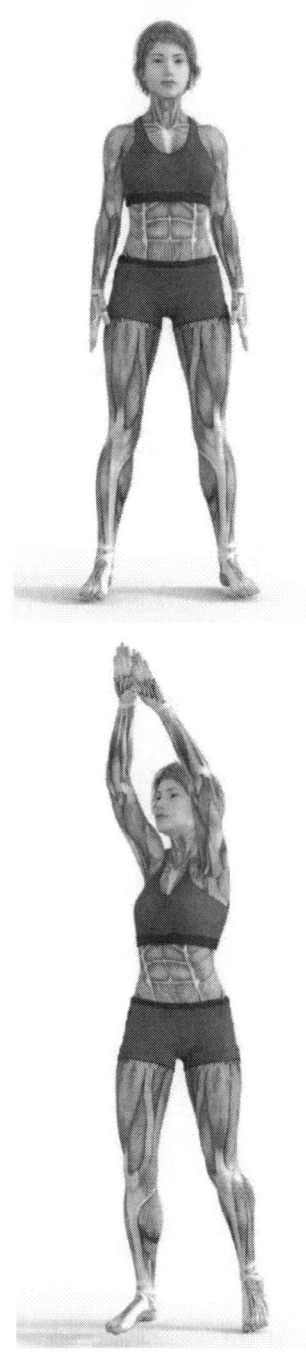

Start position

- This is a functional exercise to develop mobility of the waist, back and shoulder
- Stand with your feet about shoulder width apart, back flat and head in the neutral position
- Your arms should be straight and by your sides, palms facing inwards

Movement

- As you exhale, start to lift both arms out in front of you
- As your arms reach about chest height, start to rotate at your waist
- Continue raising your arms as you twist at the waist
- Near the top of the movement, transfer your weight slightly to the foot of the side you are rotating to
- Once at the top of movement, hold for a few seconds before returning to the start position.
- Repeat on the opposite side

Extra info

Twist and reach is an exercise that requires awareness of body position. If your shoulders are tight, you may tend to lean forward or backwards to complete the reach. If you have a mirror to check your form on this exercise, it will help identify this.

Good mornings

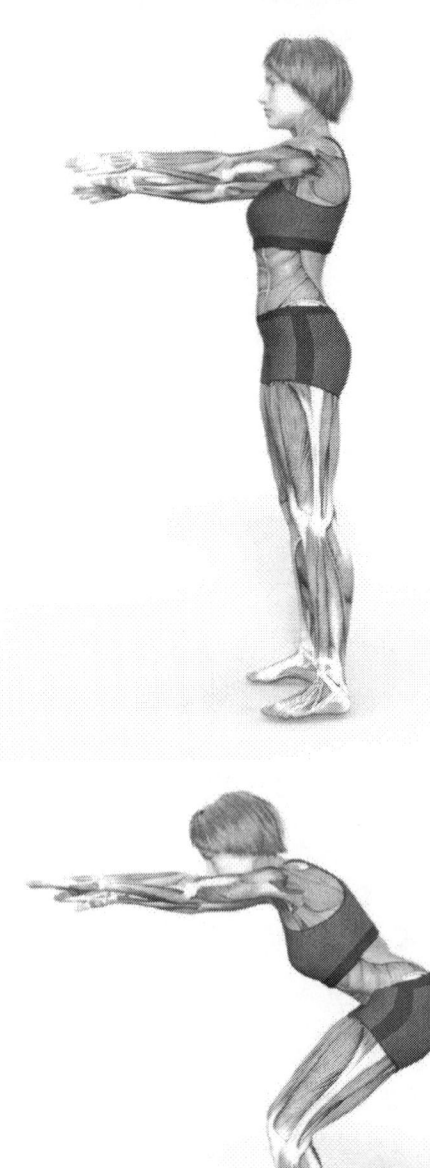

Start position

- This is an exercise to target the back and leg muscles
- Stand with your back flat, abs engaged and head in a neutral position
- Your feet should be about shoulder width apart
- Arms should be straight out in front of you and parallel to the floor

Movement

- As you exhale, start to hinge at the hips so your upper body moves forward
- Shortly after starting the hip hinge, start to bend at the knees as if you were starting a squat
- Continue both movements until your legs for a 45 degree angle from the lower to the upper and your back is almost parallel to the floor
- Once at the top of movement, return to the start position as you inhale
- Your back should remain flat throughout the exercise

Extra info

Good mornings are an excellent exercise for strengthening the hamstrings, lower back, glutes and quads, but I consider this an advanced exercise. If you would like to try this, I would recommend that you become comfortable with hip extension and squats or hover sits before adding it to your workout.

The arm position in the illustration is great for balance, but you can put your fingers on your temples or have your arms out to the sides. Whatever you choose here, you should always keep your arms in the starting position. The illustration example shows the arms always maintaining a parallel position in relation to the floor.

Lunges

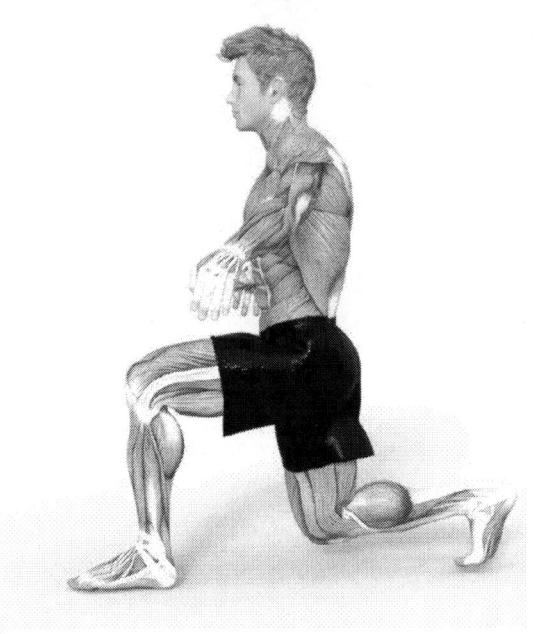

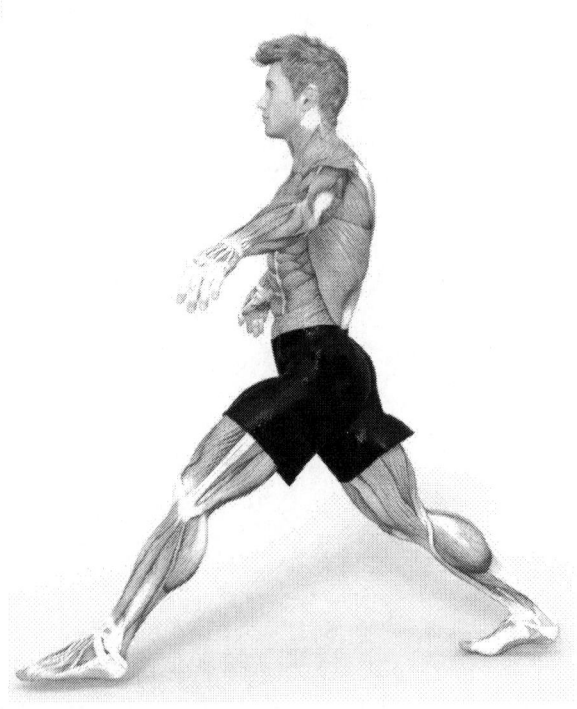

Start position

- This is an exercise to target the leg muscles
- Kneel on the floor so that your front leg forms a right angle from your calf to your hamstrings
- Your trailing leg should also form a right angle from the hamstrings to the calf
- The toes of your trailing leg should be in contact with the floor
- From this position, stand up without moving your feet position

Movement

- As you inhale, lower yourself towards the floor by bending at the knees
- Your feet should stay planted, back should stay flat and head in a neutral position
- Lower only to where the knee of the trailing leg is about to touch the floor
- Once at the top of the movement, exhale and return to the start position
- Perform a set and switch leg positions. Front leg becomes the trailing leg and vice versa

Extra info

When performing this exercise, your front knee should not move forward of your toes, this will put undue strain on the knee joints. Lunges can be performed on each leg and then the legs are switched for the second half of the set, or they can be performed as alternate lunges or walking lunges. The disadvantage here is that the setup has to be correct each time the feet are moved. More experienced trainers will have an easier time with these methods, so for new trainers to this exercise, I would advise the exercise is performed as per the description.

Squats

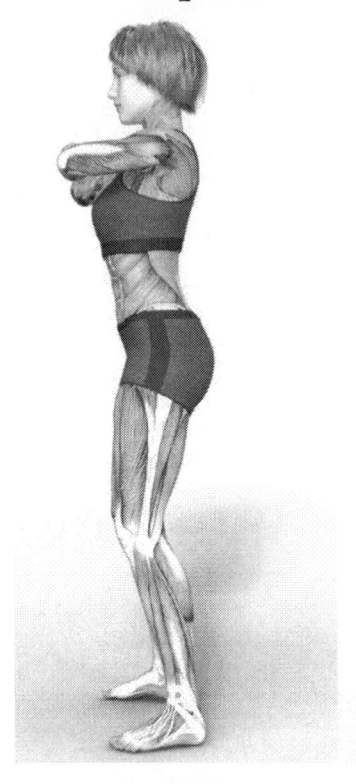

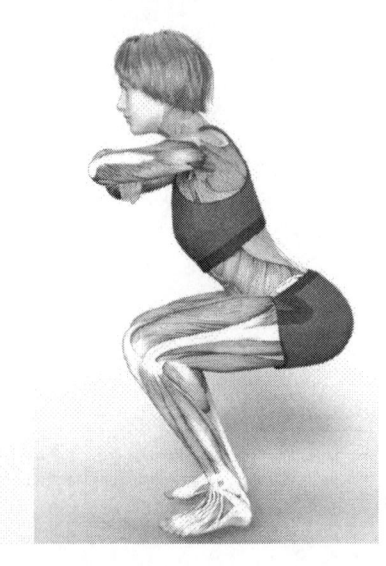

Start position

- This is an exercise to target the legs and glute muscles
- Stand with your back flat, abs and core engaged. Your feet should be about shoulder width apart and head in a neutral position.
- Fold your arms across your chest, ensuring your upper arm is parallel to the ground or have your arms straight out in front of you parallel to the ground.

Movement

- As you inhale, lower yourself by bending at the hips and knees.
- Keep your heels in contact with the floor.
- Keep your back flat, head in the neutral position and upper arms parallel with the floor.
- At the point that your quads are parallel with the floor, this is the top of movement. Once here, exhale as you return to the start position.

Extra info

This is technically the same exercise as the hover sit. The only difference is that there is no chair for reassurance and the squat is lower. The progression may seem like a subtle one, but it's significant in that being able to perform bodyweight squats without a support will give you a bigger range of movement, meaning more muscle engagement and more confidence in further progressions.

Leg lift &widening

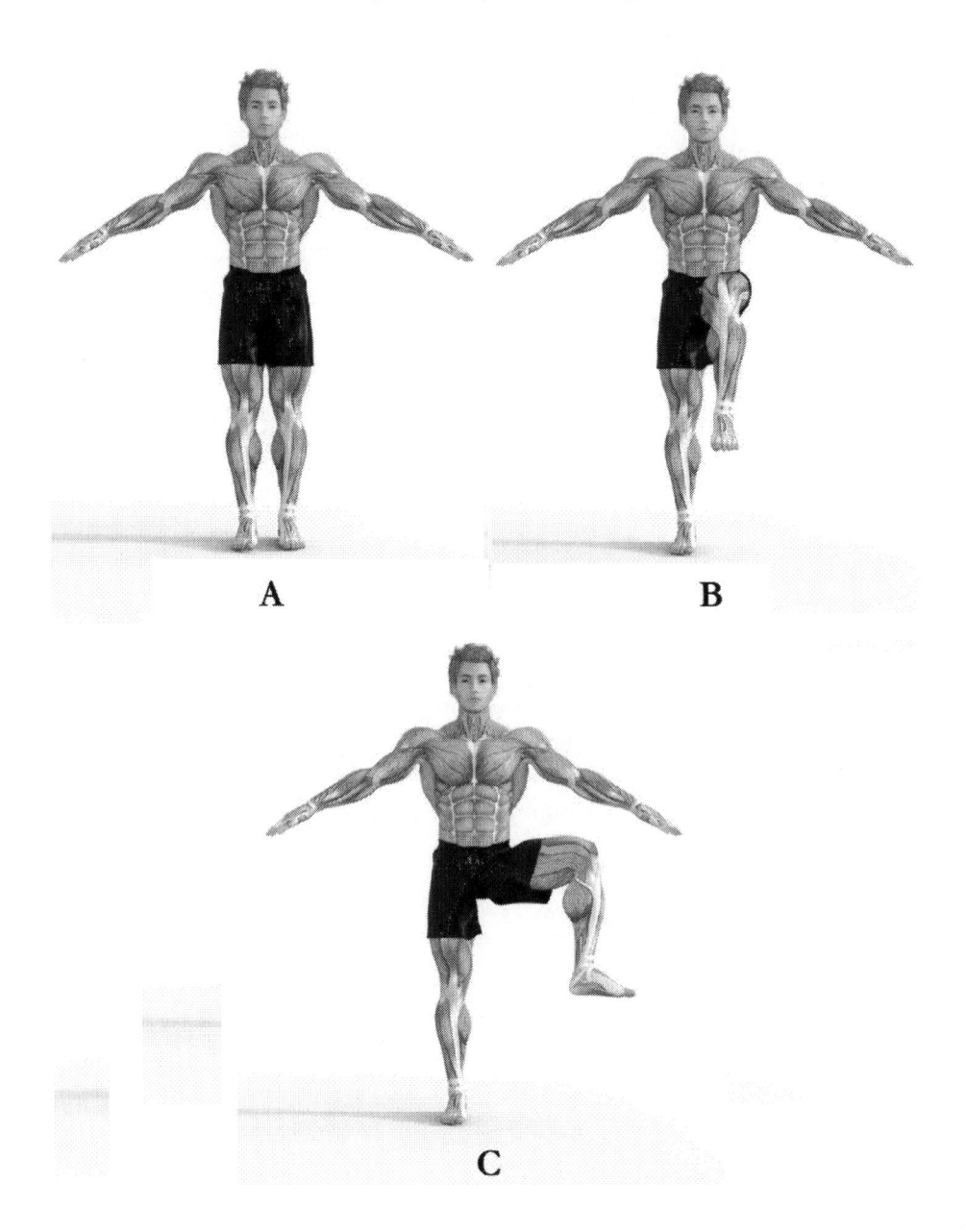

A

B

C

Start position

- This is an exercise to develop balance, quad strength, and hip mobility
- Stand with your back flat, head in a neutral position and feet close together
- Lift your arms slightly to aid with balance (A)

Movement

- As you exhale, slowly lift one leg up by extending the hip and bending the knee until your quad is parallel to the floor (B)
- Once at position B, hold for a second before bringing your leg away from your midline (C)
- Hold position C for a few seconds before reversing the movement
- Switch legs and repeat on the opposite side

Extra info

This can be very challenging for the beginner. It is still a worthwhile exercise if you cannot reach the degree of range of movement that the illustration shows. If this is too difficult, start by lifting your working leg less and also abducting your leg (taking it out to the side) less in the second part of the movement. By practicing with incremental progress with the range of movement, you will still develop stabiliser muscles and strength in these working muscle groups.

Balance & hip extension

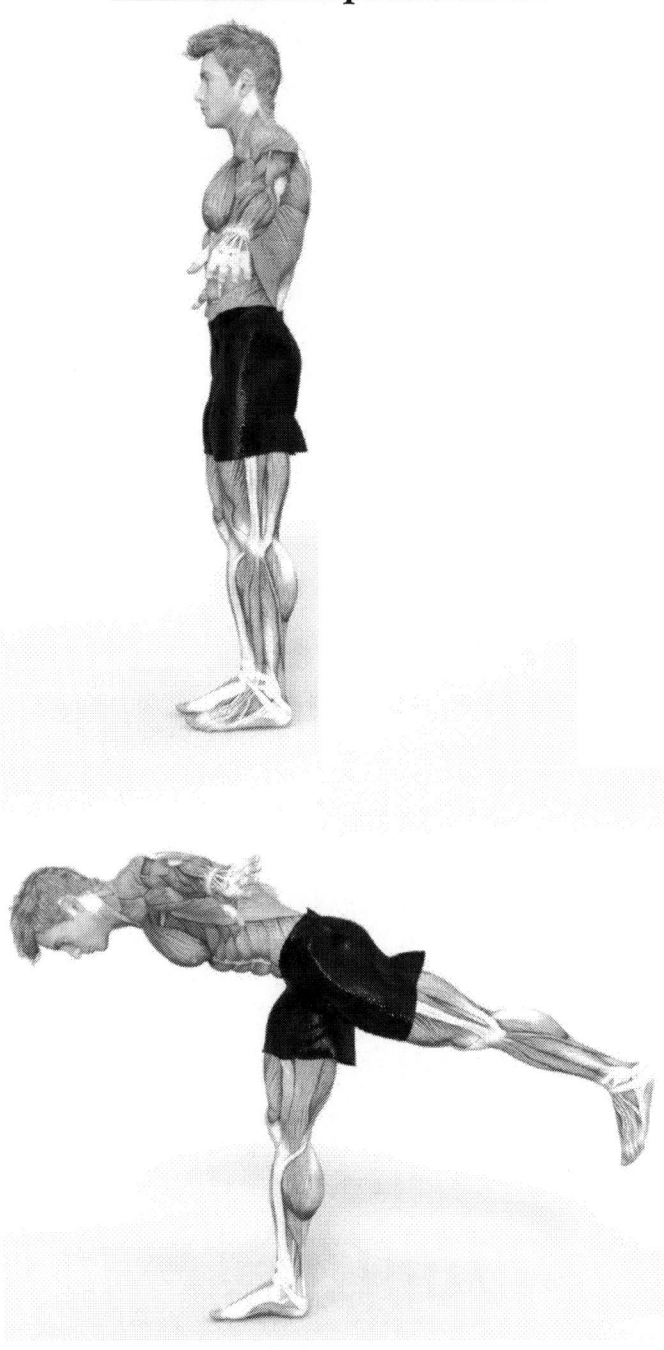

Start position

- This is an exercise to develop balance and hip mobility
- Stand with your back flat, head in a neutral position and feet close together
- Lift your arms slightly to aid with balance

Movement

- Take the weight of your body onto right leg before starting the movement
- Slowly hinge at the hip to lower your upper body towards the floor
- As you lower your upper body, start to lift your left leg to follow the line of your upper body
- Continue this movement until your upper body and left leg are parallel with the floor
- Once at the top of movement, hold for a few seconds and slowly reverse the process
- Repeat using your left leg as the load bearing leg

Extra info

As it is with the "leg lift and widening" exercise, you can still perform this movement with a limited range of motion. Progressing to where your upper body and leg are parallel to the floor can take some time, but using a smaller range of movement and practicing the exercise is a solid progression path.

Overhead push

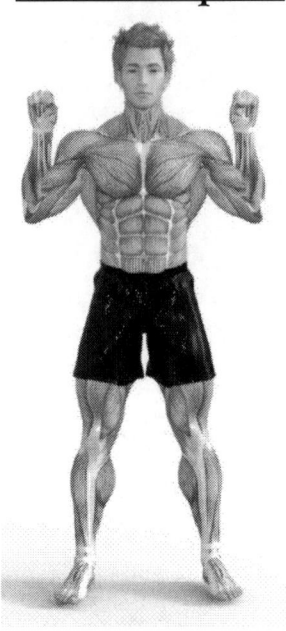

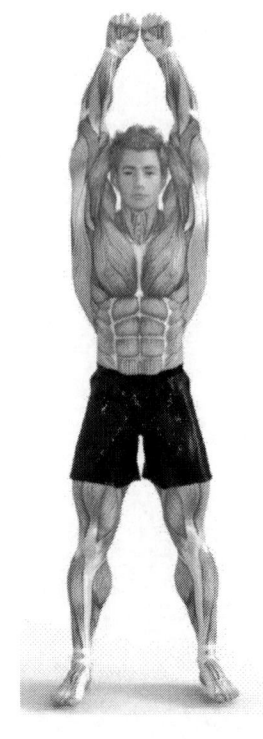

Start position

- This is an exercise to develop shoulder strength and mobility
- Stand with your back flat, head in a neutral position and feet about shoulder width apart
- Roll your shoulders backwards and lift your arms so that they are in line with your torso
- Make fists with your hands, they should be in line with your chin

Movement

- As you exhale, push your fists up above your head
- As you move your fists upwards, bring them closer together
- Try to straighten your arms directly above your head
- Once at the top of the movement, slowly and under control, inhale and return to the start position

Extra info

Like some of the other exercises in this book, this exercise can be performed with weights like dumbbells. But getting the range of movement and flexibility in the shoulders is a priority before moving onto workouts with resistance.

When pushing your fists above your head, be aware of their position. A common mistake here is to move the fists and arms forward of the head. This will neglect the rear shoulder muscles slightly and dilute the value of the exercise.

Chest opening & push

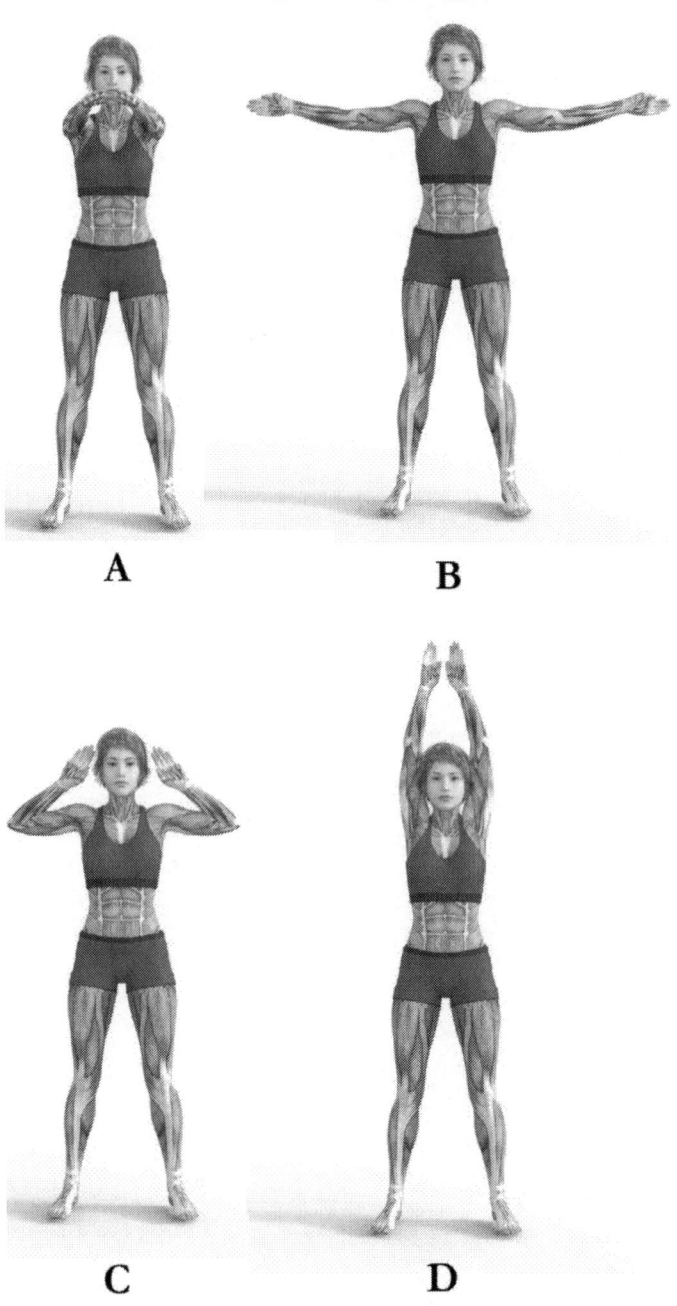

A

B

C

D

Start position

- This is an exercise to develop mobility in the chest and shoulders
- Stand with your back flat, head in the neutral position and feet about shoulder width apart
- Straighten your arms and raise them out in front of your upper torso. They should be parallel with the floor and palms facing downwards (A)

Movement

- Slowly and under control, bring your arms out to your sides, maintaining their height, whilst twisting your palms until they are facing directly forward. Continue the movement until you feel a stretch across your chest. Hold this position for a few seconds (B)
- From position B, bend at the elbows so that your fingers make contact with the sides of your head (C)
- From position C, push your hands directly above your head until fully extended (D)
- Hold position D for a few seconds before slowly returning to the start position

Extra info

Believe it or not, holding your arms so they are parallel with the floor is actually work that challenges your shoulder muscles, so if you maintain this alignment, through a full set of this exercise, you will probably feel a slight burning in your shoulders. The push from position C to D will engage all three muscles further.

Remember to keep a flat back throughout the exercise and to push your hands directly above your head.

Bent over row

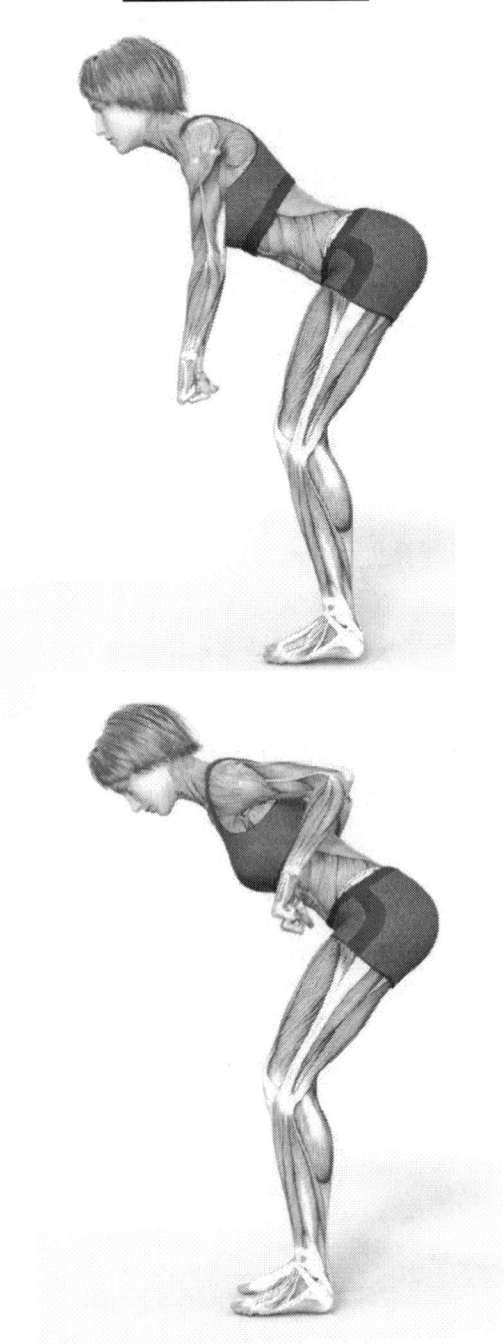

Start position

- This is an exercise to target the back muscles
- Your hands should be about shoulder width apart and palms facing back. Making fists will help here
- Straighten your arms but keep a slight bend in the elbows
- Bend your knees slightly
- Keep your back flat and hinge at the hips so your upper body is set at about 45 degrees to the floor
- Your arms should hang in down in front of your upper torso

Movement

- As you exhale, pull your fists towards your belly button
- Keep your back flat and glutes engaged
- Focus on pushing your chest forward and your shoulders back
- Keep your elbows towards your body's midline
- Inhale as you return to the start position

Extra info

It is possible to perform this exercise with your upper body at a right angle to the floor, but in my experience, this puts more strain on the lower back, so 45 degrees is preferable. When bringing your fists towards your body, remember to maintain a flat back.

Pick & lift

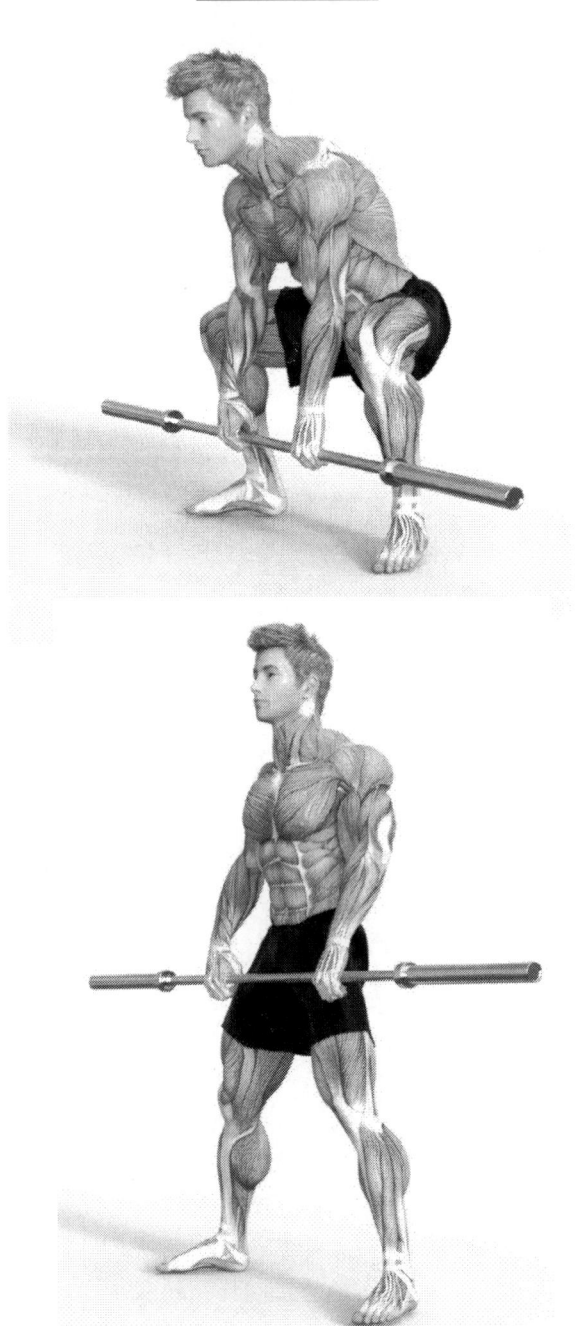

Start position

- This is an exercise for the back and legs
- Select an object that has an even weight distribution and stand with your toes either side of it
- Your toes should be in line with your knees
- Squat down and take and grip the object with both hands. Your hands should be inside your knees
- Keep your back flat and head in a neutral position
- Your feet should be flat on the floor

Movement

- Before you lift, ensure that your elbows are slightly bent and locked in this position
- Engage your glutes and abdominals
- As you exhale, stand up with the object, keeping it close to your body and pull your shoulders back
- Once at the top of the movement, inhale and return to the start position

Extra info

This is technically a "deadlift". I've chosen to use an illustration showing a weight lifting bar as the object to be lifted. If you don't have a bar, a broom handle is a good place to start. You can also use other objects like a small tin or even something like a football, you can even perform this movement without an object at all.

This is a big movement that challenges the function of a whole range of muscle groups and I would advise that becoming comfortable with bodyweight squats first, before adding this one to your workouts.

Weight swing

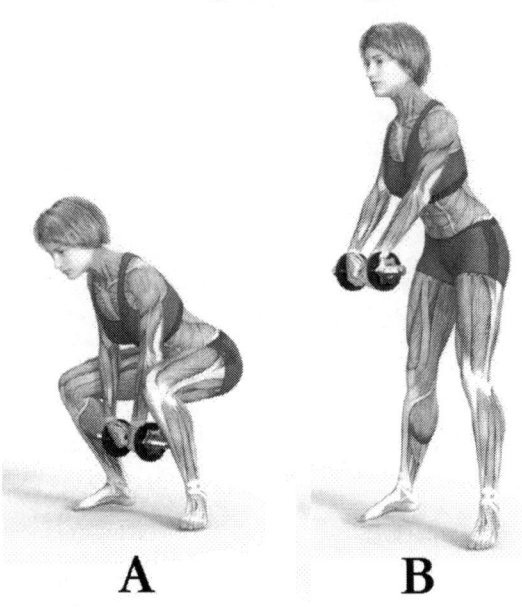

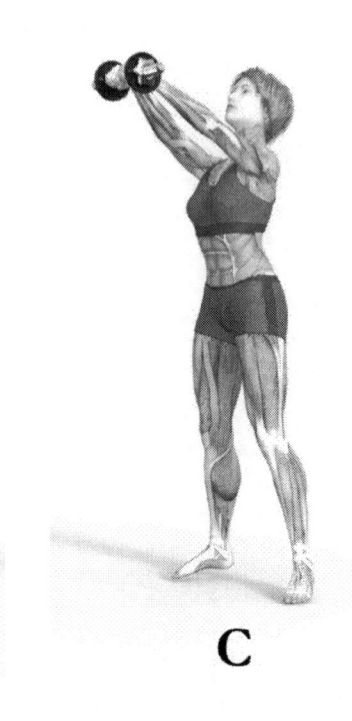

A

B

C

Start position

- This is an exercise for the back, legs and shoulders
- Select an object that has an even weight distribution and stand with your toes either side of it
- Your toes should be in line with your knees
- Squat down and take and grip the object with both hands. Your hands should be inside your knees
- Keep your back flat and head in a neutral position
- Your feet should be flat on the floor (A)

Movement

- Before you lift, ensure that your elbows are slightly bent and locked in this position
- Engage your glutes and abdominals
- As you exhale, stand up with the object, keeping it close to your body and pull your shoulders back (B)
- Once at position B, raise the object to just above head height. At the top of the movement, your back should be flat and arms fully extended (C)
- Once at the top of movement, reverse the process to finish at position A

Extra info

Although this is called a "weight swing", we are not actually using momentum to swing the weight. The exercise should be performed slowly and with control. I consider this an advanced movement as there are a lot of muscle groups involved, so I'd advise becoming comfortable with squats and the pick and lift exercises before adding this to your workouts.

Again, the object used does not have to be a dumbbell. It can be anything that's got an even weight distribution and is easy to grip. Of course, this exercise can be performed with no object at all.

Cross leg sit

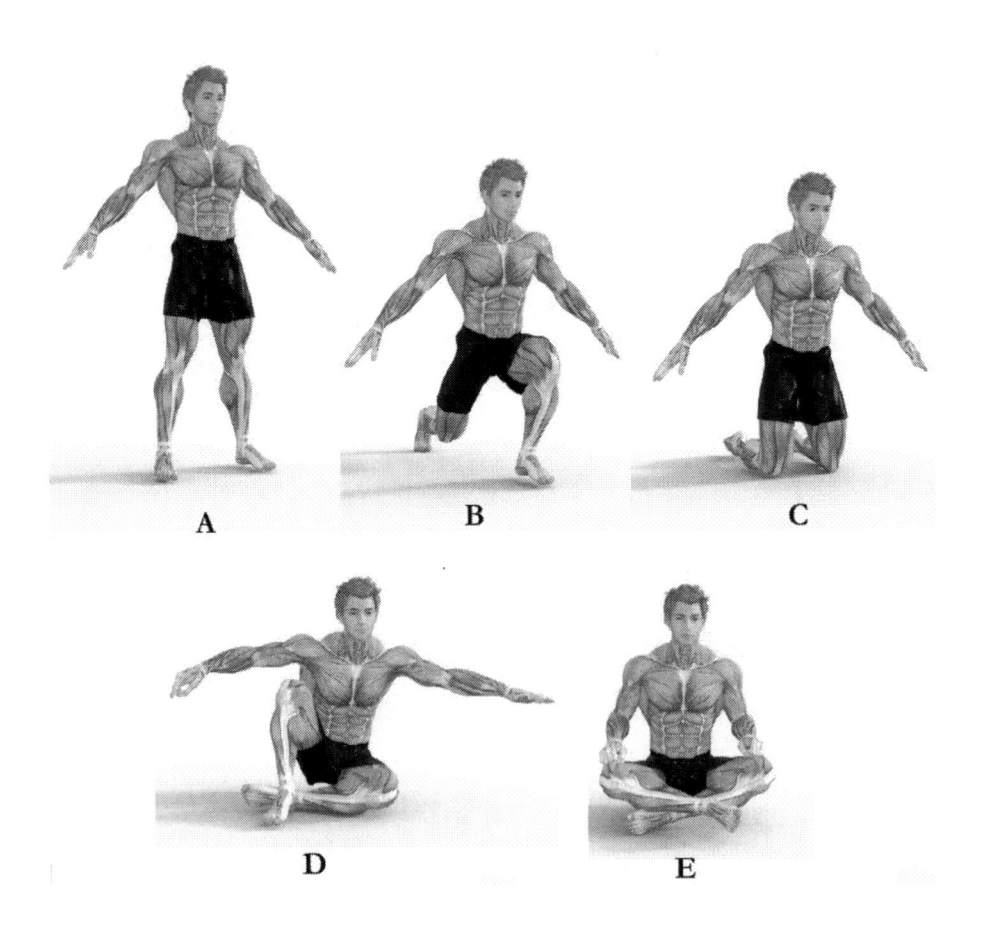

A

B

C

D

E

Start position

- This is an exercise to develop balance, core strength and hip and leg mobility
- Stand with your back flat, head in a neutral position and feet about shoulder width apart (A)

Movement

- Take a step forward and slowly kneel until one of your knees is taking your bodyweight (B)
- Whilst maintaining a flat back, draw the leading leg backwards to align with your kneeling leg. Your bodyweight should now be going through your knees (C)
- Slowly and under control, sit back onto your lower legs and transfer your weight from the front of your lower legs to the left
- Move your right leg forward and away to place your right foot onto the floor, bring your left leg forward and transfer your weight to your left glute (D)
- Finally, cross your legs and maintain a flat back (E)
- Hold this position for as long as you are comfortable and reverse the process

Extra info

Getting into a cross leg position on the floor without using your hands can be tough, and holding the position can be just as tough for some.

If you would like to do this exercise but have not yet developed the flexibility and strength, try going through it stage by stage and working up this way. For example, if kneeling down is challenging, practice this part of the exercise until you can do it, then move on to the next stage.

Thank you! If you found this useful I'd like to help further...

First off, I would like to thank you for your purchase. It really means a lot that you chose to spend your time on this guide. I am a self-published author with a passion for training and helping people get to where they want to be with fitness and by reading; you are supporting me and fuelling my passion.

This guide should give you a brilliant start into the world of functional training and the planning and prep that goes with it. But this is not my first fitness book! I've been writing and self-publishing for several years. I've written books on fitness motivation, planning, resistance band training, bodyweight exercise, bodybuilding, home workouts and long distance running. These guides are based on my experience and formal education.

I've been a long distance endurance runner, a competing bodybuilder, and I have worked with personal training clients to change their lives through fitness, so I have a lot to share.

If you found this short guide useful and would like to read more about body transformations, fitness motivation, home workouts or more about resistance training and would like a clear path to follow, I have plenty more for you to look at including workbooks and journals for you to plan and track!

Most of my books are available in eBook and paperback format, and some are also available as audio titles narrated by an awesome voice actor called Matt Addis.

Each fitness book is written as a standalone guide but also has its place as part of a series. So if you are a total beginner and want to become a bodybuilder or marathon runner as an end goal, I have you covered! Jump in at the start of the series with **"Fitness & Exercise Motivation"** and follow the steps, I'll be at the starting blocks with you and we will cross the finish line together!

If you would like to learn more about this series and my other books, you can do so by visiting my author page. Visit Amazon and search "James Atkinson", you will see my ugly mug, click it, and you'll be taken to my page.

As we all know, diet plays a big part in health and fitness, and the two subjects fit hand in hand. So I would like to offer you a free download of seven healthy recipes that I created and use regularly myself. You can copy the recipes exactly, add your own twist to them, or simply take inspiration from them.

If you would like to grab this along with other free content such as video tutorials, motivation and fitness planning guides become a part of my email list and we'll reach our fitness goals together! You can do so by following the link below, or using the QR code.

https://yourfitnesssuccess.com/all-the-freebiees/

Don't worry, I never spam, and newsletters are infrequent, but there is always something of value inside when they are sent.

Thanks again, I wish you all the best!

Cardio training.

I'd like to leave you with this excerpt from one of my other books *"Marathon training & distance running"*.

Cardio training can range from walking to running, from jogging to circuit training and intervals, so it's a pretty broad subject that wears many faces! Adding some form of cardio is always recommended for everyone. A regular, short, brisk walk can make the world of difference to some.

This book is not about cardio training, but I know for a fact that fitness training can be positively life changing. Cardio is part of fitness and just happens to be the most accessible form of exercise for most people. Walking, jogging, running and sprinting are activities that most of us can get stuck into right away.

Before I was a bodybuilder, I was a long-distance runner and before I was a long-distance runner; I was a cardio failure! The journey from cardio failure to long distance endurance runner was a life changing one for me and I learned a lot from this, so much so that I wrote a bestselling book on the subject.

I want to share a part of this with you now. Here is an excerpt from the book. I hope you enjoy it and find it useful.

CHAPTER 7 - Marathon Training & Distance Running

WHERE TO START

This section is really aimed at the beginner, but it may still hold some useful information for the veteran.

With anything that you do, you have to start from the beginning, and I firmly believe that having a solid foundation to build on is a must if you want results.

It would be great if every goal that you had was achievable overnight, but with any serious fitness goal, the mind-set of progression training is a fundamental factor for success!

Of course, you would not expect to be able to run a marathon in a few short weeks of training. And I would like to clarify that if you are just starting out, there is a long road ahead of you… (Excuse the pun.)

This may sound negative, and many people would be put off by the fact that at least six months of hard, consistent, and smart training will only get them a small step closer to their goal.

I'm talking about the guys that have never done any exercise before and would like to take up the challenge of a marathon.

If you are this guy or gal, I would first like to congratulate you on making this decision and also like to reassure you that you CAN do this.

When you cross that finish line, I'm sure that it will be one of the greatest accomplishments of your life, and your training, character building, and determination leading up to this accomplishment will definitely enrich you as a person.

YOUR FIRST RUN (WHAT TO EXPECT)

The first time you step out of your door, you will probably be motivated, have some shiny new running shoes and training attire, and be ready to start pounding the pavement.

There are a few things that can literally kill your motivation and make you hang up your new running shoes permanently if you are not careful. The biggest killer of your goals in this situation is...

"too much, too soon."

I have seen it, overheard conversations about it, and actually been there myself.

Everything's great. You are all ready to start your marathon training, you have planned your route, you are hydrated, and you know this is going to be the start of something very special! You give a few cursory hamstring stretches and set off on your first run.

Two minutes in and you are fighting for air, your lungs are on fire, you feel sick, and you are wondering how on god's green earth you are even going to finish your first run when you are in this state and you can still see your front door?

Believe me; if you have never felt this way before, you need to actually be there to understand the mental effect that this has on you. It can be devastating!

You will no doubt be able to relate to this feeling very soon as your training progresses. But I will say that it can be controlled, and when you look back at these events, they won't seem that bad. It's just while you are there that you will feel your world is ending!

Before you start your training, please read the Breathing and Running Style chapters. If you can understand and practice this before you even start your first run, it will help you out massively.

YOUR FIRST RUN (WHAT TO DO)

Once you have your breathing and running style sorted, you will be ready for your first run.

The thing is, your first run will not actually be a run! Remember that this is all about progression and you have to start somewhere. If you have never been on a run before, your body isn't used to the kind of stresses put on it, so you will probably end up in the state that we just talked about.

Once you have your route planned out, you should don your trainers and get ready, as you would expect. But your first training session should be a steady walk around your route. This will benefit you more than you probably think.

First of all, it will start you on your routine. Next, it will get you used to your new running shoes. These are a vital piece of kit for any runner.

"Bad shoes = Bad feet, and with bad feet, you can't do a whole lot of running"

Another thing that walking your route will help you with is getting your body used to prolonged activity. These early sessions will also help you to prepare mentally for your training too as you will be able to visualise your route and you will get to know how long this will take you or how close you are to the finish line.

Depending on how fit you are or how quickly you progress, you may want to do this walk for the first full week, but you can assess your progress after your first session.

All that being said, starting off slowly is one thing, but progression is vital if you want to improve and actually reach "long-distance runner status."

This "easy start" approach may be refreshing to some readers, but you also need to progress and push yourself. It may take you a few weeks to find your limits and assess your fitness progression, but this is all part of the process. It is important that you find the right balance.

This is what I would do if I had never done any fitness:

First Session

- Walk my route at a consistent pace

Second Session

- If the previous session was too easy, I would pick up my pace a bit.

- If the previous session was too hard, I would shorten the route a bit.

- If the previous session made me out of breath slightly and had me sweating but I was otherwise comfortable, I would consider a short jogging stint at the last section of my next session.

As you can see, there are a few factors that you can change each time that you train. The important part at this stage is to never sit back and go through the motions; you MUST be progressing. If your sessions do not push you slightly, you will not develop the endurance that you are looking for.

But at this point, there is no need to get to the stage of physical discomfort mentioned at the beginning of this chapter. It will only mess with your mind.

Also by James Atkinson

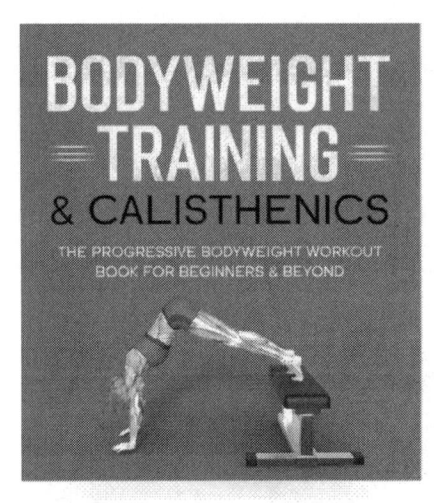

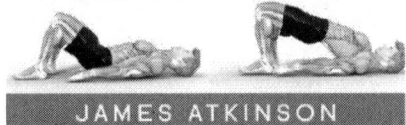

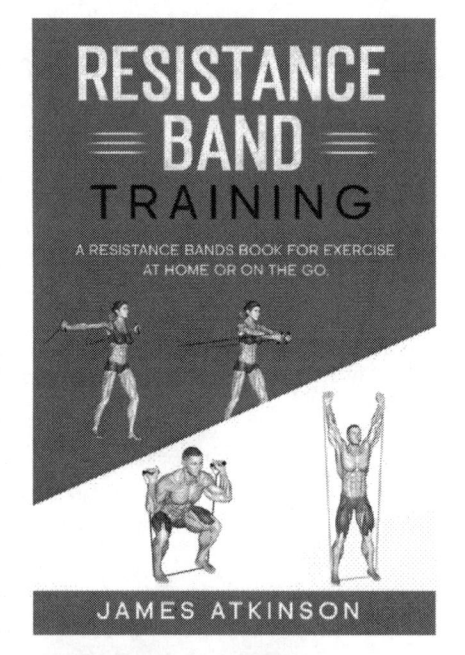

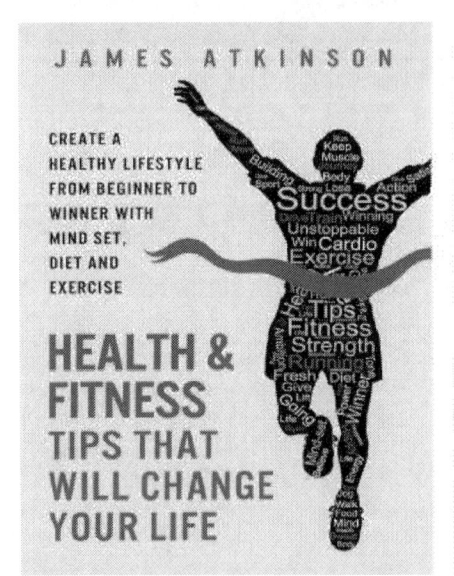

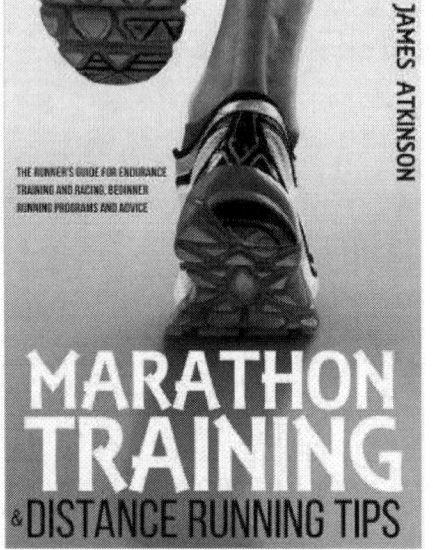

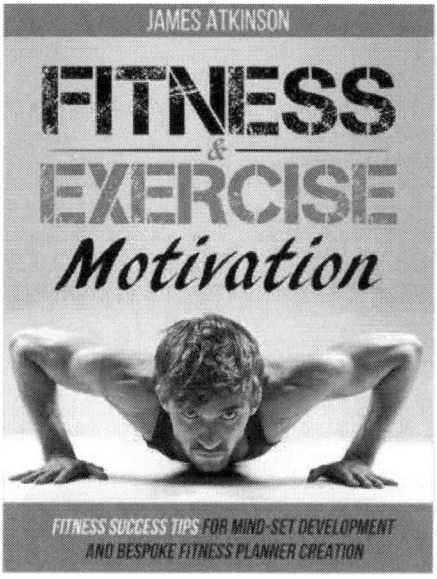
JAMES ATKINSON
FITNESS
&
EXERCISE
Motivation
FITNESS SUCCESS TIPS FOR MIND-SET DEVELOPMENT
AND BESPOKE FITNESS PLANNER CREATION

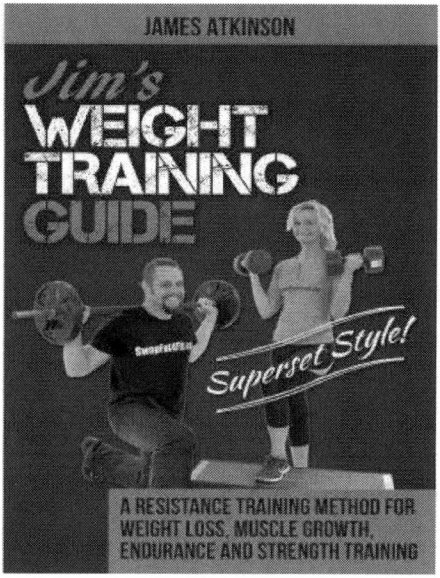
JAMES ATKINSON
Jim's
WEIGHT
TRAINING
GUIDE
Superset Style!
A RESISTANCE TRAINING METHOD FOR
WEIGHT LOSS, MUSCLE GROWTH,
ENDURANCE AND STRENGTH TRAINING

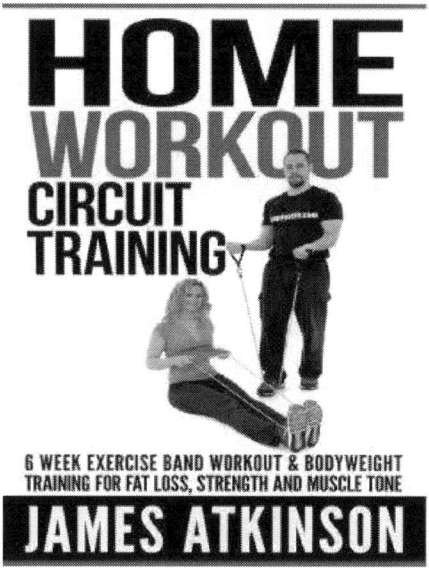
HOME
WORKOUT
CIRCUIT
TRAINING
6 WEEK EXERCISE BAND WORKOUT & BODYWEIGHT
TRAINING FOR FAT LOSS, STRENGTH AND MUSCLE TONE
JAMES ATKINSON

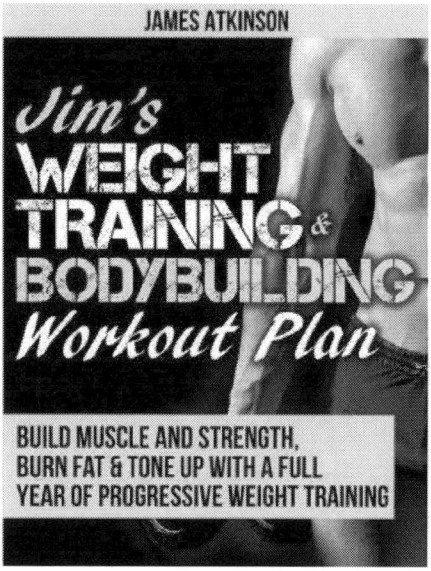
JAMES ATKINSON
Jim's
WEIGHT
TRAINING &
BODYBUILDING
Workout Plan
BUILD MUSCLE AND STRENGTH,
BURN FAT & TONE UP WITH A FULL
YEAR OF PROGRESSIVE WEIGHT TRAINING

Blank workout cards

FUNCTIONAL TRAINING			
ROUTINE			
EXERCISE	SETS	REPS	TIME

WEEKS	MON	TUE	WED	THURS	FRI	SAT	SUN
1							
2							
3							
4							
5							

FUNCTIONAL TRAINING

ROUTINE	

EXERCISE	SETS	REPS	TIME

WEEKS	MON	TUE	WED	THURS	FRI	SAT	SUN
1							
2							
3							
4							
5							

FUNCTIONAL TRAINING

ROUTINE	

EXERCISE	SETS	REPS	TIME

WEEKS	MON	TUE	WED	THURS	FRI	SAT	SUN
1							
2							
3							
4							
5							

FUNCTIONAL TRAINING

ROUTINE	

EXERCISE	SETS	REPS	TIME

WEEKS	MON	TUE	WED	THURS	FRI	SAT	SUN
1							
2							
3							
4							
5							

YOURFITNESSSUCCESS.COM

PUBLISHED BY:

JBA Publishing

http://www.yourfitnesssuccess.com

admin@yourfitnessuccess.com

Functional Exercise For Seniors

Copyright © 2022 by James Atkinson

All Rights Reserved.

No part of this book may be reproduced or transmitted in any form or by any means, electronic, mechanical, photocopying, recording, or otherwise, without prior written permission of James Atkinson, except for brief quotations in critical reviews or articles.

Requests for permission to make copies of any part of this book should be submitted to James Atkinson at admin@yourfitnessuccess.com

DISCLAIMER

Although the author and publisher have made every effort to ensure that the information contained in this book was accurate at the time of release, the author and publisher do not assume and hereby disclaim any liability to any party for any loss, damage, or disruption caused by errors or omissions in this book, whether such errors or omissions result from negligence, accident, or any other cause.

First published in 2022

Printed in Great Britain
by Amazon

d6400379-3768-42ac-83d2-08a7135caa96R02